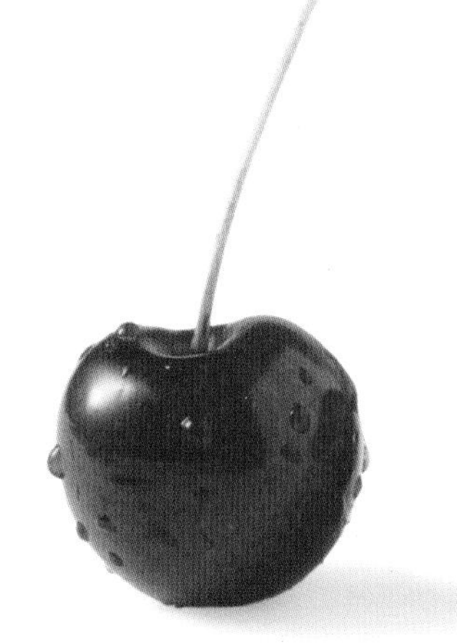

In bed with The Food Doctor

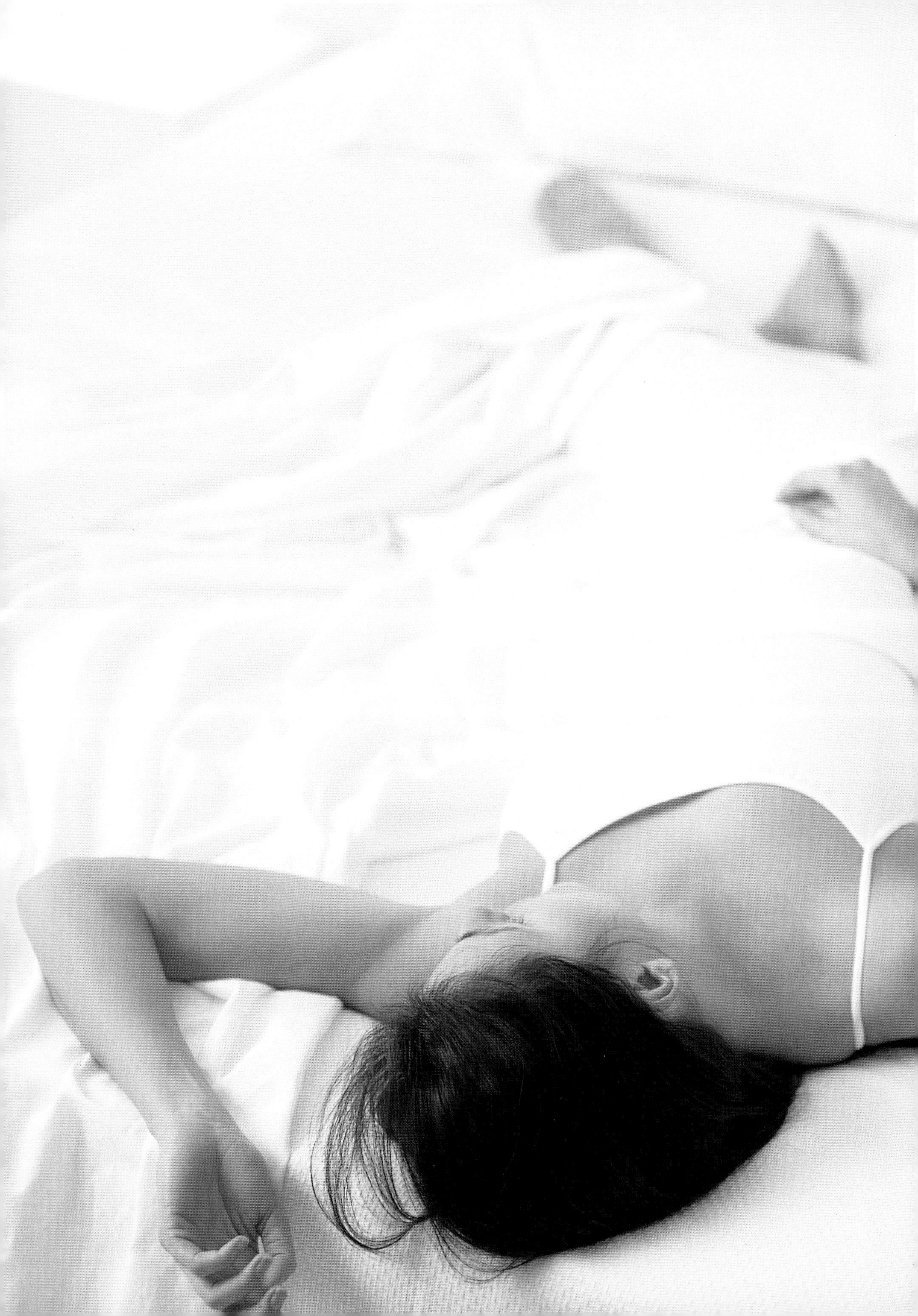

In bed with
The Food Doctor

HOW TO EAT YOUR WAY TO BETTER SEX AND SLEEP

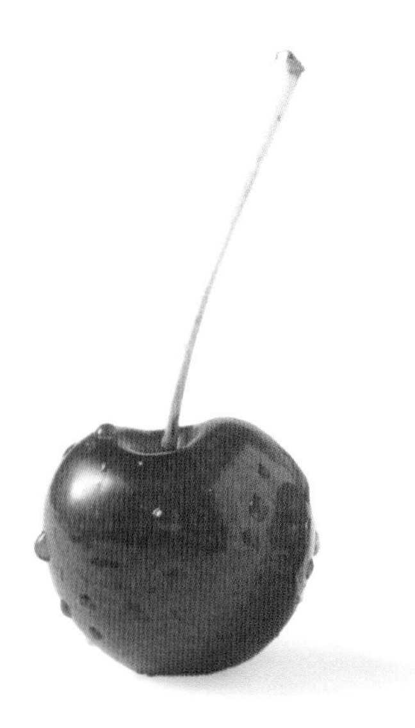

Ian Marber Dip ION & Vicki Edgson Dip ION

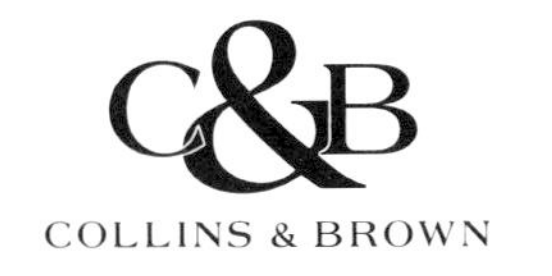

For Johnathon
Ian

For Wayne
Vicki

The author's grateful acknowledgements go to Nellie Piggott for her excellent preparation of the recipe section, to Juliet Dennis for her inexhaustive research, to Michael da Costa for believing in us and to Antonia Smith for her unending support.

The publishers would like to thank the following people for their help with this book: XAB Design; Ian O'Leary, for the food photography; Neil Mersh, for the photographs of the people in bed; Catherine Lewis, Judy Bugg, Mandy Greenfield, Annie Lee and Margaret Binns.

First published in Great Britain in 2001 by
Collins & Brown Limited
London House
Great Eastern Wharf
Parkgate Road
London SW11 4NQ

Distributed in the United States and Canada by
Sterling Publishing Co., 387 Park Avenue South, New York, NY 10016, USA

9 8 7 6 5 4 3 2 1

British Library Cataloguing-in-Publication Data:
A catalogue record for this book is available from the British Library

ISBN 1 85585 899 1

Commissioned by Grace Cheetham
Art directed by Anne-Marie Bulat
Project managed by Clare Churly
Edited by Mandy Greenfield
Designed by XAB Design
Photography by Ian O'Leary, Neil Mersh and Catherine Lewis

Reproduction by Classic Scan Pte Ltd, Singapore
Printed and bound in Singapore by Craft Print International Ltd

This book was typeset using Helvetica and DIN.

Safety Note
The information in this book is not intended as a substitute for medical advice. Any person suffering from conditions requiring medical attention, or who has symptoms that concern them, should consult a qualified medical practitioner. All nutritional supplements should be taken under the supervison of a qualified nutritional practitioner.

contents

sex

sleep

Sex and sleep – in an ideal world they would both occur naturally, yet there are many factors that can influence the quality of both. We spend approximately one-third of our lives in bed – sleeping, dozing and making love – but we pay little attention to the functional and physiological aspects of this very important part of our lives. Many of us are familiar with sleep-related issues, such as insomnia, but sexual problems are perhaps the ultimate taboo. Even in this age of discussion and openness few people will admit that they are experiencing problems of a sexual nature.

Problems in both areas are common, however, and often have relatively simple remedies. A change in lifestyle, the addition or avoidance of certain foods or food groups, and cutting out stimulants are all steps that can make a difference. However, very little has been written about either subject from a nutritional standpoint, so we felt it was time to redress this.

We spend approximately one-third of our lives in bed – sleeping, dozing and making love.

It has long been acknowledged that correct nutrition plays a powerful role in overall health. However, the level of nutritional information available recently has become confusing for many people. All too often the properties of one nutrient are trumpeted and promoted to such an extent that many of us decide to take that nutrient in supplement form and await a miracle. But it must be remembered that nutrients work synergistically – that is, more productively together than in isolation – so increasing a single nutrient will not always produce the desired effects.

We should always examine the underlying cause of each health issue and work to rebalance the body accordingly. For example, if you suffer from insomnia, taking melatonin at night might help you fall asleep, but it will not do anything to help explain why insomnia has become a problem. The sleepless nights might be indicative of other issues and taking a sleep remedy might mask the symptoms. The same is true of sexual dysfunction. While taking Viagra may overcome the immediate problem, the cause has not been addressed.

In Bed with The Food Doctor examines problems in the areas of both sex and sleep, highlighting potential causes and explaining how nutrition can be a powerful remedy.

introduction

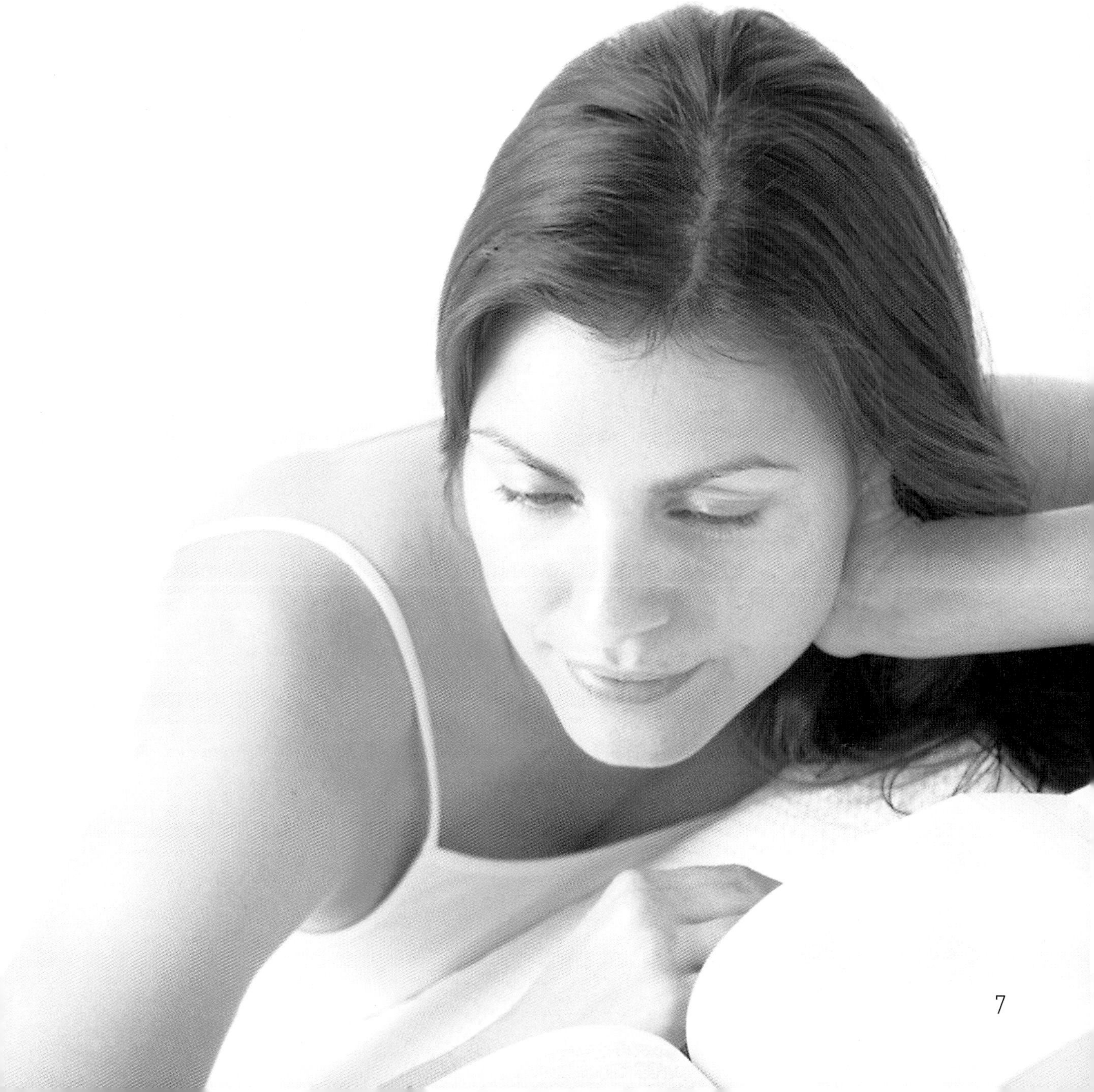

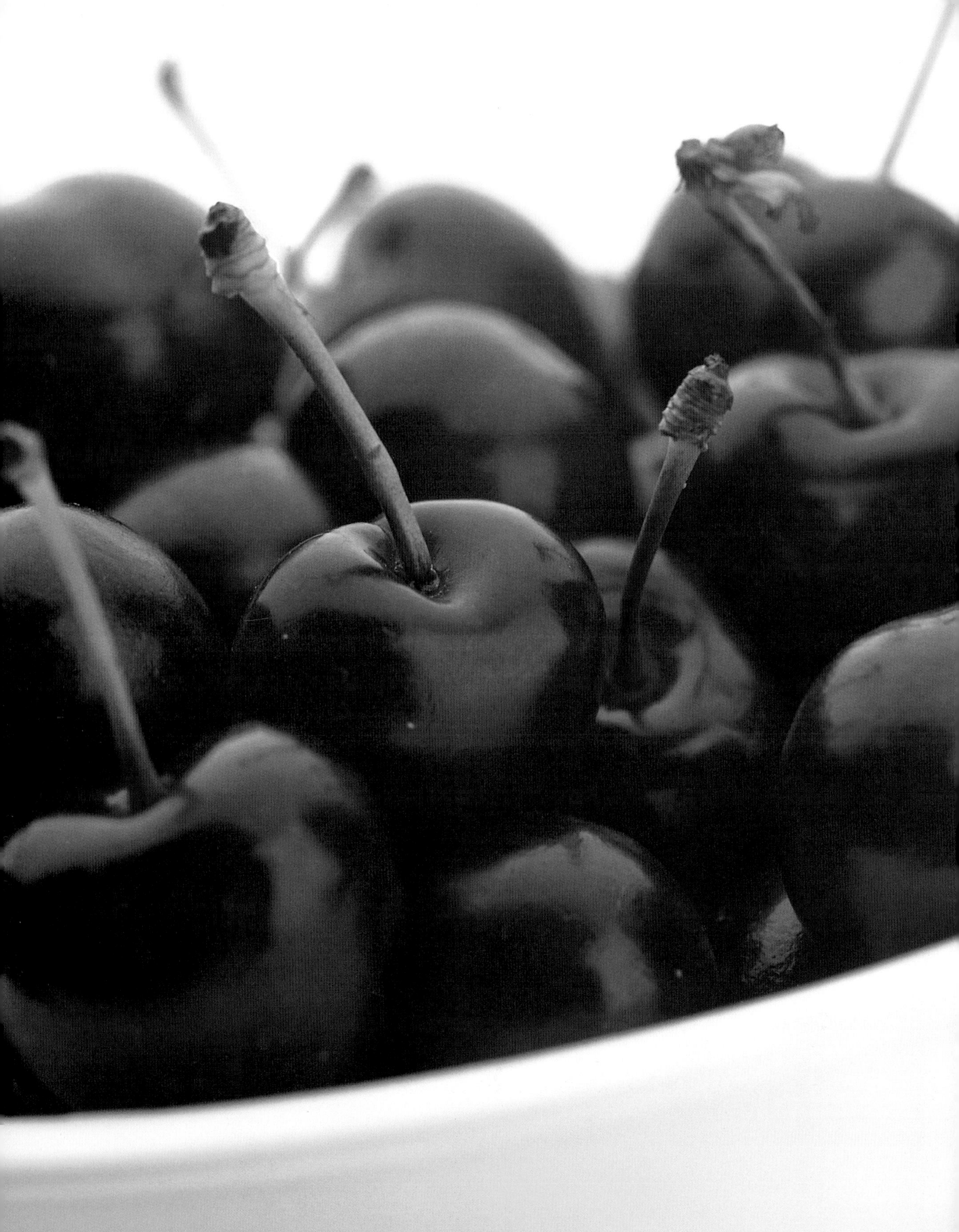

PART ONE: **SEX**

sex

foods to boost

your sex life

why sex is go

All animals have an inborn instinct to seek out a mate in order to reproduce, but humans are perhaps the only mammals that involve their emotional well-being in the physical act, employing the senses of sight, taste, touch, smell and sound, both as a form of stimulation and as a means of relaxation.

The 'feel-good' factor

As well as giving physical pleasure, the sexual act has several specific benefits. It is known that endorphins – hormone-like compounds that are released during physical stimulation and exertion (including pain) – actually create a feeling of well-being within us. These natural pain-relievers are targeted on certain sites in the body, namely the spinal column, the pituitary gland at the base of the skull and the testes, and they create a sense of relaxation, enhanced mood and increased sensitivity to touch.

We all know that we enjoy it, and why we indulge in it, but do we actually know what sex can do for us?

Those of us who have experienced the benefits of a good massage are well aware that there are several areas of the body that are more sensual than others – these areas tend to occur where endorphin receptor sites are most abundant. This is one of the reasons why massage and foreplay are both seen as catalysts for satisfactory sex, as some people are less easily stimulated than others and these actions help to promote the release of 'feel-good' endorphins.

It is interesting to note that chocolate contains a chemical called theobromine that boosts endorphin production, thus partly explaining the appeal of this potentially addictive food. Endorphins target opiate receptors on the cell membranes in the brain for their potential pain-relieving properties, inducing a sense of pleasure – and chocolate behaves in the body in the same manner as opiate drugs, albeit to a lesser degree. Perhaps this explains why so many brands use seductive product names and images in their advertising.

Immune stimulation

It has been found that regular, satisfying sex also boosts certain immune cells, known as natural killer cells, that are among the most abundant of the immune cells circulating in the body. They are

od for you

stimulated by endorphins and by a hormone called oxytocin, which is released from the pituitary gland in the brain. These killer cells are responsible for keeping potentially damaging viruses, bacterial infections and rogue-cell development (such as that of cancer cells) under control, so sex may also help to keep illness at bay.

Calorie control?

There has been much speculation as to whether or not sex is an adequate form of exercise on its own. Although some sexual positions do tend to require more stamina and strength than others, it has been shown that the average length of sexual activity burns up relatively few calories. It would take several hours of strenuous sex to have a substantial effect on calorie reduction. Looking at this from another angle, it is more beneficial to tone up the body and increase your stamina and cardiovascular health in the gym to ensure a healthy and active sex life at home!

The pleasures of sex

Notwithstanding the physical benefits of sex, there is also the small question of pleasure. Sex is an intimate part of any relationship and creates a sense of emotional and physical well-being. Chemical reactions in the body occur to make this happen. For instance, levels of the hormone oxytocin rise by up to 500 per cent during sex, which, in addition to increasing immunity, will induce drowsiness and relaxation after the sexual act, ensuring a good night's sleep.

Another chemical present during sex, known as PEA (phenylethylamine), creates the feelings of light-headedness and light-heartedness, and is chemically similar to amphetamine, which explains its addictive quality. Interestingly, this compound is used to create many man-made stimulants and anti-depressants, as it has a direct effect on the levels of dopamine (a neurotransmitter that regulates mood, see p. 49) in the brain.

So we can see that sex is good for us for a number of reasons, many of which we shall look at in more detail later on. First, we address the issue of why and when our appetite for sex becomes reduced, and what we can do about such problems. Look at the questionnaire on pp. 12–15 to establish which areas of your life may be affected by your sexual appetite.

sex questionnaire

Look through the following questionnaire, then take some time answering the different sections. Not all areas will apply to everyone, and some of the questions may seem irrelevant to you. However, we have found that most sexual inhibitions and problems arise from a combination of emotional and physical factors, and it may surprise you to learn how great a part our environment plays in our total sexual health.There is no scoring system – the questionnaire is simply designed to raise your awareness of the different factors that can affect your sexual appetite and pleasure, so that you know which of the sections that follow will be most applicable to you.

GENERAL HEALTH AND FITNESS

Most of us wish we could be in better health than we are, knowing that our fitness levels equate with our sexual stamina and libido. Take a look at how well you really are. Many of the problems outlined here relate to lowered immunity.

1. Do you suffer from frequent colds and infections?
2. Have you often taken antibiotics for these problems?
3. Do you suffer from recurrent bouts of fatigue and lack of energy?
4. Do you have any allergies or intolerances?
5. Do you have asthma/hay fever/eczema?
6. Do you bruise easily?
7. Are your wounds slow to heal?
8. Do you have recurrent digestive problems?
9. Do you experience frequent headaches/migraines?
10. Do you suffer from athletes' foot, thrush or cystitis?

STRESS

Stresses come in many shapes and forms, and affect all areas of our lives, in particular our libido. Read through the following questions to identify which particular stresses may be affecting you.

1. Do you find it difficult to relax when you have time off?
2. Do you never manage to take time out each day from your busy schedule?
3. Are you always 'on the run'?
4. Do you carry out several tasks simultaneously?
5. Are you competitive by nature?
6. Do you lose your temper easily?
7. Do you often forgo exercise due to fatigue or a hectic schedule?
8. Do you fly long-distance more than once a month?
9. Do you suffer from insomnia?

HEART HEALTH

A healthy heart allows us to enjoy rigorous exercise without undue exertion or effort, affording us a strong libido and sexual appetite. Unfortunately our lifestyles and eating habits often impede optimum heart health, leading to fatigue and shortness of breath.

1. Have you experienced angina or severe heart pain recently?
2. Do you find yourself short of breath after climbing stairs?
3. Are you less fit than you used to be?
4. Is your blood pressure higher than 120/75?
5. Do you take regular exercise that raises your heartbeat for more than 20 minutes?
6. Do you have cold hands and feet?
7. Do you have poor circulation?
8. Do you suffer from varicose or thread veins?
9. Do you experience palpitations?
10. Do you add salt to your food?

ERECTILE DYSFUNCTION

There are several causes of erectile dysfunction (see p. 52). In many cases these problems can be rectified, and it is important to see a doctor if you have been experiencing erectile dysfunction for some time.

1. Are you over 45 and, if so, have you had a Prostate-Specific Antigen (PSA) test in the last year (to examine contributory factors, such as swollen prostate)?
2. Do you urinate more frequently than you used to?
3. Are you unable to maintain an erection for any length of time?
4. Do you experience discomfort during intercourse?
5. Do you experience pain or a burning sensation when urinating?
6. Have you noticed a decrease in the level of seminal fluid production?

TOXICITY

A number of toxins affect our libido and general vitality. Some of these toxins may have been stored in our bodies for years and take their toll by affecting our energy production.

1. Do you smoke more than five cigarettes daily?
2. Do you drink alcohol daily?
3. Have you indulged in recreational drugs for a number of years?
4. Are you on any prescription medication?
5. Do you have amalgam fillings in your teeth?
6. Do you live in a busy, built-up area?
7. Are you excessively exposed to car and transport fumes?
8. Do you work in the airline industry?
9. Did you grow up on an agricultural farm?

HORMONE DISRUPTION

Hormones are chemical messengers that control our body functions, and some hormones are intricately linked to sex, so that a hormone imbalance (see p. 00) can have widespread repercussions on our enjoyment of the sexual act.

FEMALE

1 Are you currently taking the contraceptive pill?
2 Do you suffer from severe premenstrual syndrome (PMS)?
3 Have you had any form of fertility treatment?
4 Have you suffered a miscarriage in the last three years?
5 Are you on any medication for hormone regulation?
6 Do you suffer from breast tenderness?
7 Is there a history of breast/ovarian/uterine cancer in your family?
8 Do you suffer from irregular menstruation or have you experienced amenorrhoea (cessation of regular menstruation) at any time?
9 Do you have an excessive growth of body hair?
10 Have you had breast implants?

MALE

1 Are you experiencing hair loss or a receding hairline?
2 Has your weight distribution increased around your abdomen?
3 Do you have a noticeably lower sex drive than you used to?
4 Have you noticed any unexplained weight gain over the last few years?
5 Are you currently taking any medication for hypertension, any anti-depressants or tranquillizers?
6 Has the production of your body hair or facial hair changed?
7 Have you had any hormone treatment (such as testosterone patches)?
8 Have you taken steroid medication for asthma, eczema or other inflammatory conditions for more than two years?

DIETARY FACTORS

Good diet plays a major part in our overall health, but it is also a contributory factor to hormonal balance, cardiovascular health and regulated energy production, which, as we will see, plays an important part in enhancing sexual desire.

1 Do you consume a lot of processed, ready-prepared meals?
2 Do you eat fried food regularly?
3 Do you eat red meat more than twice a week?
4 Do you suffer from constipation or flatulence?
5 Do you take antacid medication for indigestion?
6 Do you consume more than two cups of tea/coffee per day?
7 Do you drink more than two units of alcohol daily?
8 Do you occasionally experience feelings of bloatedness?
9 Is your diet rich in dairy produce?
10 Do you often consume canned carbonated drinks?

DEPRESSION

There are varying grades of depression (see p. 47), all of which inevitably have an effect on sexual interest and libido. One of the first signs of low-grade depression is, in fact, a noticeable loss of interest in sexual activity.

1. Are you unclear about certain goals in your life?
2. Have you lost interest in socializing with other people?
3. Do you spend a lot of time on your own out of choice?
4. Do you set tasks for yourself that you find it impossible to complete?
5. Have your sleep patterns become disturbed?
6. Have you recently lost weight, or lost your appetite?
7. Have you become tearful for no specific reason?
8. Do you feel overwhelmed with your life at the moment?

FATIGUE

There are many understandable causes of fatigue (see p. 51). However, if there appear to be other causes of fatigue that you have not yet sorted out, this may be having a direct effect on your libido.

1. Do you wake in the morning still feeling tired?
2. Does even mild exercise exhaust you?
3. Do you have less energy now than you used to?
4. Do you feel that you need to go to bed early at night?
5. Does your body feel heavy at any time during the day?
6. Do find that you lose concentration and focus in the latter part of the afternoon?
7. Have you suffered recently from a virus from which you have not yet fully recovered?

BLOOD-SUGAR MANAGEMENT

How we digest and absorb our food is the key to our production of energy throughout the day. Fatigue is the second most common cause (after stress) of lack of interest in sex, so understanding how you regulate blood-sugar management (see p. 40) is important.

1. Do you suffer from bouts of fatigue throughout the day?
2. Do you have frequent sugar and caffeine cravings?
3. Do you often have an unquenchable thirst?
4. Do you easily become irritable or angry?
5. Do you tolerate others poorly?
6. Do you feel fatigued towards the end of the day?
7. Do you wake up feeling the need for more sleep?
8. Do you sometimes feel dizzy and light-headed?
9. Are you prone to fainting?
10. Is there a history of diabetes in your family?

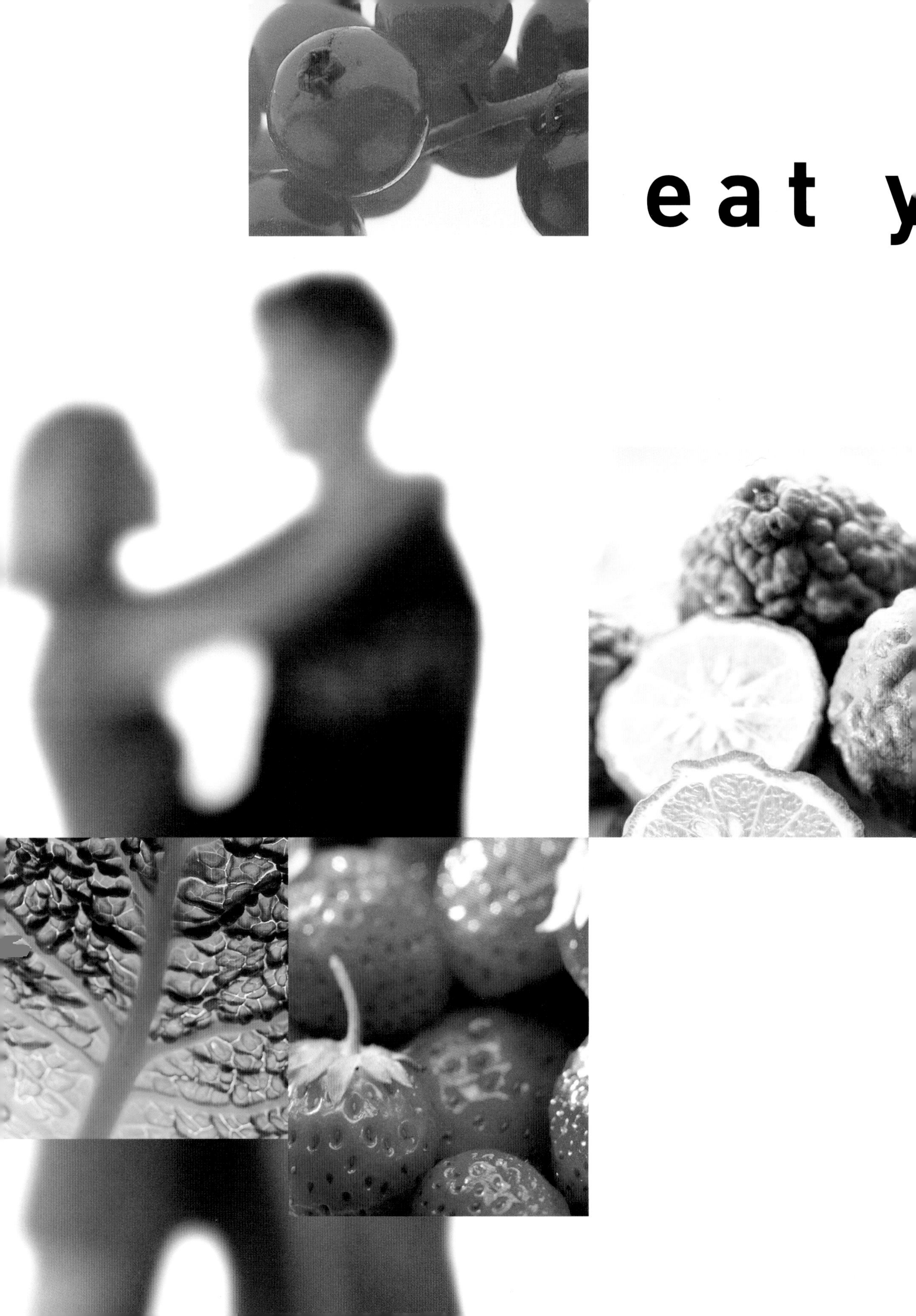
eat y

our way to better sex

foods to improve the quality of your sex life

It is important to understand which factors control our sex life. The equilibrium of our sex hormones is the primary factor, but this is intimately linked to our metabolic hormones, which control our growth and cell repair, our immune, digestive and respiratory systems.

All nutrients are required for optimum health yet some are more linked to sexual health and function than others. In this section we have identified the most important of these nutrients, together with their richest sources.

There are certain basic principles that apply to increasing libido and sexual pleasure. Skipping meals or overeating will inevitably lead to fatigue and therefore we espouse eating little and often throughout the day. One vital key to enhancing stamina ultimately lies with optimum blood-sugar management (see p. 40).

Another equally important area to address is the limiting of the long term damage that can result from stress. This is done through the support and nourishment of the relevant stress glands with appropriate nutrition.

The following pages explore specific nutritional deficiencies and illustrate the everyday foods that we can include in our diets to allow us to eat our way to better sex.

nutritional deficiencies

There are numerous symptoms that indicate particular nutrient deficiencies, but there are also some very specific minerals and vitamins that are required for sexual health and reproduction. Look at each of the following groups of questions separately; if you answer 'yes' to three or more questions in any one group, then it is possible that you are deficient in that mineral or nutrient.

IRON	FUNCTION	RICHEST SOURCES
• Do you tire easily? • Do you have pale skin? • Do you get out of breath easily? • Do you feel dizzy after mild exertion? • Are cuts and wounds slow to heal? • Do you suffer from heavy periods?	**Iron** is required for the formation of haemoglobin in blood, which carries oxygen to every cell in the body for energy production; this is needed for the process of arousal and the sexual act. Iron is essential for the absorption of vitamin C, which must be consumed daily, because it cannot be stored by the body.	Liver, red meat, chicken, caviar, raisins, prunes, apricots, egg yolks, wholegrains, watercress, spinach, broccoli, beetroot (beet) and pulses, although the body absorbs animal-based iron sources more readily than vegetable sources. 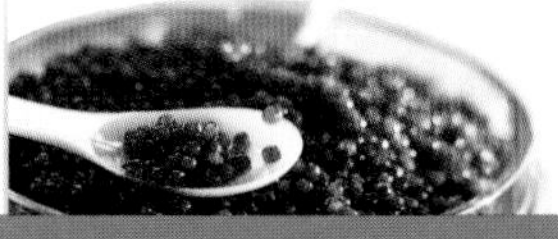

ZINC	FUNCTION	RICHEST SOURCES
• Do you have stretch-marks? • Do you get frequent infections? • Does a cut or wound take a long time to heal? • Do you have any white flecks on your fingernails? • Do you have difficulty tasting food? • Do you add salt to your food? • Do you have a poor sense of smell? • Do you find some smells excessively offensive? • Have you suffered from infertility problems? • Do you have premature hair loss or early-greying hair? • Do you suffer from confusion or memory loss? • Do you get eczema or psoriasis?	**Zinc** is undoubtedly the most important mineral for sexual behaviour and fertility. The tail of the sperm is formed from zinc, giving it its motility (ability to swim/move), and zinc is vital for adequate sperm production and healthy semen (each ejaculation holds approximately 5mg of zinc). It is also required for the formation of all enzymes that govern taste and smell, which are required for sexual arousal. It is needed in large quantities at puberty for the development of sexual organs and is essential for all growth and reproduction.	Shellfish and seafood (particularly oysters and sardines), eggs, cheese, lamb, chicken, turkey, liver, steak, brown rice, lentils, pine nuts, pumpkin and sesame seeds, spirulina and wholegrains. 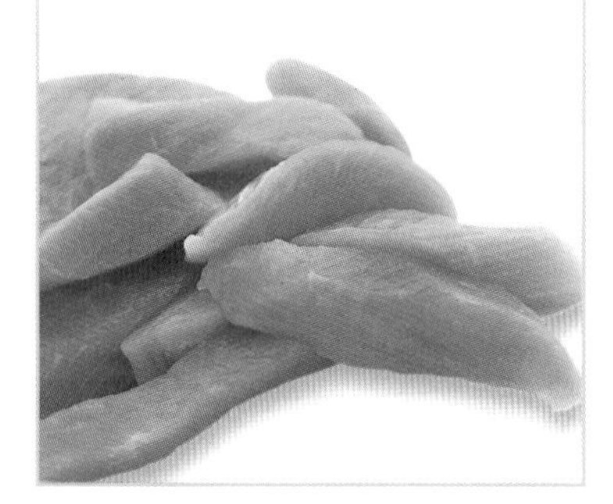

MAGNESIUM	FUNCTION	RICHEST SOURCES
• Do you get muscle cramps? • Do you have sleep problems? • Are you easily startled? • Do you have problems relaxing? • Do you suffer from bad menstrual cramps? • Do you experience muscle weakness, tiredness or pain? • Do you become easily fatigued? • Do you suffer from anxiety? • Are you suffering from osteoporosis?	**Magnesium** is required for the absorption of calcium, and most Western diets are higher in calcium than magnesium, because of our prolific consumption of dairy produce. This mineral is also essential to balance the sex hormones and regulate the muscle contraction and relaxation of the heart. It is needed for the production of energy, so it plays a very important role in sexual stamina. It is also vital for sexual sensitivity, arousal, ejaculation and orgasm.	Green leafy vegetables, nuts, cheese, bananas, cereal grains, caviar and seafood. 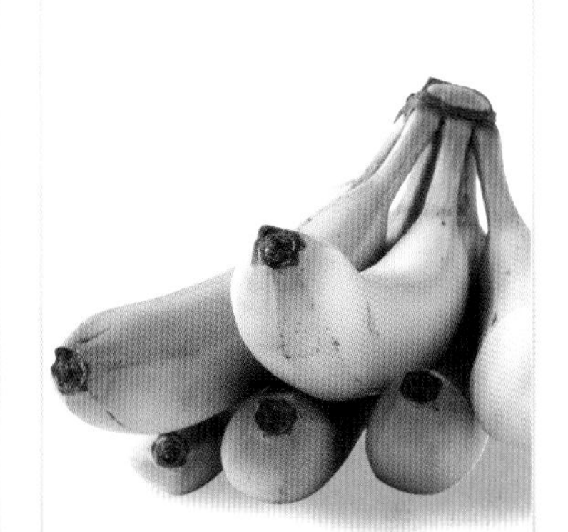

CALCIUM	FUNCTION	RICHEST SOURCES
• Do you suffer from insomnia? • Are you nervous and jumpy? • Do you experience tingling sensations in your arms or legs? • Do you occasionally have muscle twitches? • Do you have poor dental health? • Do you suffer from arthritis? • Do you ever experience heart palpitations?	**Calcium** is essential for cardiovascular health and for bone strength and growth. It also plays a part in nerve transmission, enabling the sensation of touch to be arousing. It is required for the muscle contraction associated with the male erection and female orgasm. It is also a component part of all bodily fluids.	Dairy products, green leafy vegetables, beans, beetroot (beet), watercress, prunes, nuts, dried fruit, shellfish and small fish that are eaten whole (e.g. sardines and whitebait). 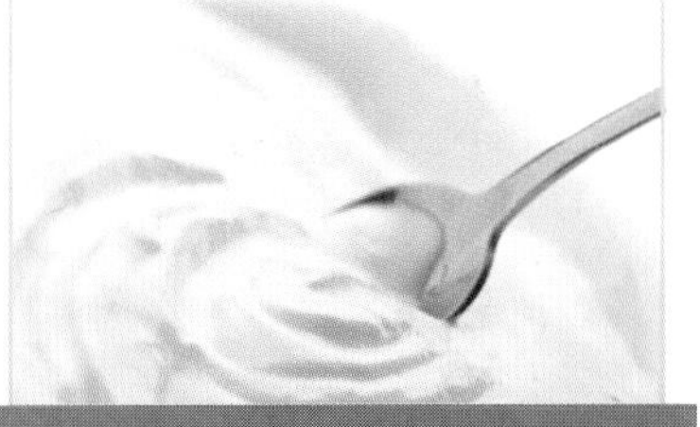

IODINE	FUNCTION	RICHEST SOURCES
• Are you constantly tired? • Do you have cold hands and feet? • Do you cry easily? • Do you suffer from puffy skin? • Do you have a slight swelling of the neck at the throat? • Have you lost your appetite? • Have you lost your mental alertness? • Have you gained weight inexplicably?	**Iodine** is needed to produce thyroxine to stimulate the thyroid gland, which is the organ that regulates metabolism and energy production and produces hormones. Poor thyroid function inevitably leads to loss of libido (see p.54 and 59).	Shellfish and seafood, kelp and other seaweeds (particularly blue-green algae), spirulina, watercress, Swiss chard, turnips and their greens, squash, watermelon, cucumber, spinach and okra.

SELENIUM	FUNCTION	RICHEST SOURCES
• Do you suffer from frequent infections? • Do your wounds heal slowly? • Is there a family history of cancer? • Do you tire easily? • Are you suffering problems of infertility?	**Selenium** is essential for the immune system, for protection against infections and in the utilization of oxygen, which is required for stamina. It has also been linked to the regulation of sex drive, sperm count and fertility. Some countries show very poor soil levels of selenium, so supplementation may be necessary to provide adequate quantities if you suffer from poor sex drive or lowered fertility.	All shellfish and seafood, sesame and pumpkin seeds, Brazil nuts, butter, liver and kidney. 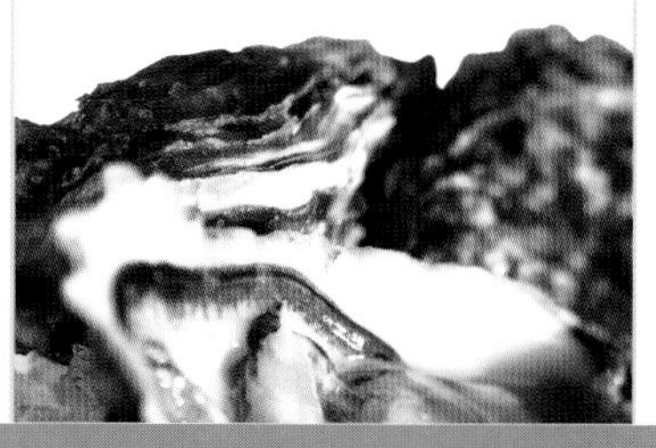

CHROMIUM	FUNCTION	RICHEST SOURCES
• Do you feel tired after eating? • Do you become irritable if you don't eat regularly? • Do you suffer from cold hands and feet? • Do you sometimes feel dizzy for no apparent reason? • Are you always thirsty? • Do you need to urinate frequently?	**Chromium** is vital for efficient utilization of insulin, which regulates blood-sugar levels, and for energy production by carrying circulating blood glucose to the cells. Fast and ready-made foods adversely affect blood-sugar levels, placing an increasing burden on the pancreas to produce insulin in ever-increasing quantities. From a sexual perspective, a deficiency of chromium in the diet will affect energy levels and subsequently libido.	Soya products, brewers' yeast, cucumbers, onions and garlic. 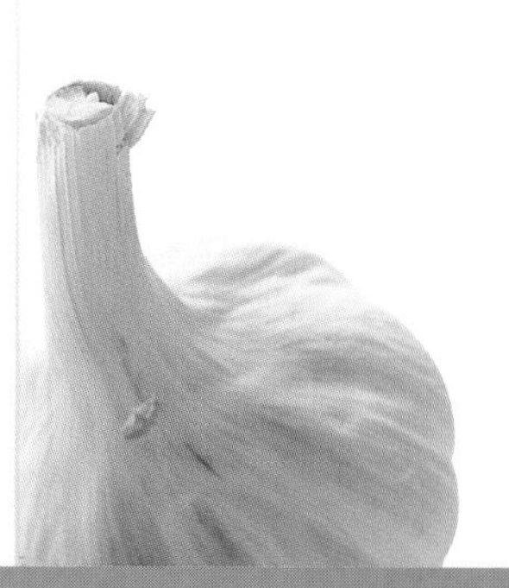

ARGININE	FUNCTION	RICHEST SOURCES
• Do you tire easily? • Do you suffer from anorexia or bulimia? • Has your adult growth been slow? • Do you suffer from poor or unsatisfactory ejaculation? • Do you heal slowly?	**Arginine** is an amino acid that is derived from protein foods. It is required for all growth and sexual development and is the main component of the head, or body, of the sperm, so it is essential for healthy sperm production.	All animal foods, dairy products and popcorn (which has the highest level of vegetable-based arginine). 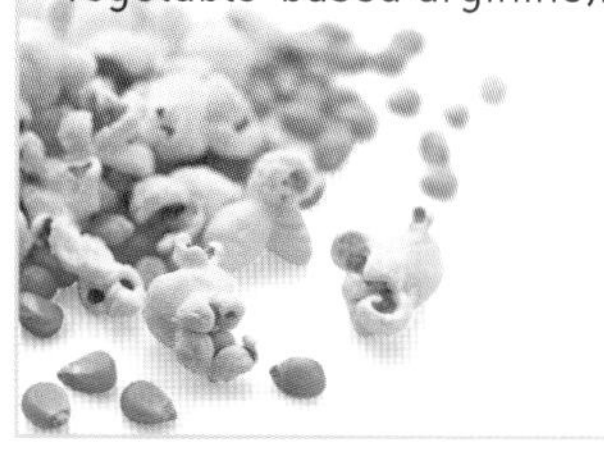

CO-ENZYME Q10	FUNCTION	RICHEST SOURCES
• Do you suffer from constant fatigue? • Do you experience heart palpitations? • Are you tired after exercise? • Do you suffer from short bursts of energy followed by fatigue? • Do you feel unrested upon waking? • Do you easily become breathless after mild exertion? • Do you suffer from 'lead legs'?	**Co-enzyme Q10** is a nutrient required specifically in the end-stage of energy production at a cellular level. It is needed by every cell in our body, where small power-houses, known as mitochondria, produce and release the energy that we use on a moment-by-moment basis. Co-enzyme Q10 production declines with age, although our demand for it does not.	All animal foods, spirulina, blue-green algae and chlorella (all 'green foods': vegetarian sources of potent proteins), spinach, sardines and peanuts. 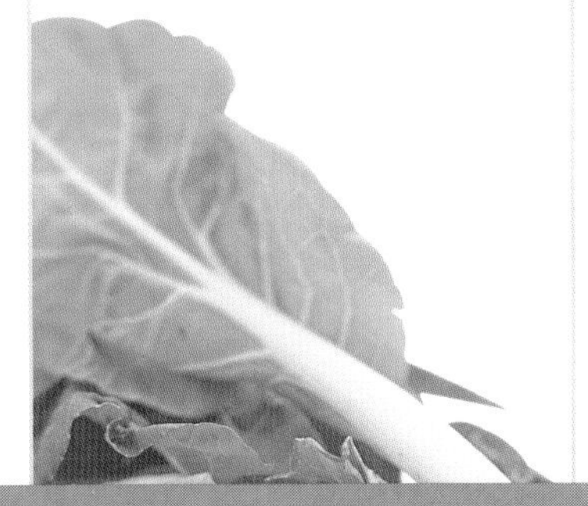

ESSENTIAL FATTY ACIDS	FUNCTION	RICHEST SOURCES
• Do you suffer from dry skin? • Do you have stretch marks? • Do you have small bumps or spots on the back of your upper arms? • Do you have cracked nails, dry hair or peeling lips? • Do you have thickening of skin on the heels? • Are you prone to PMS? • Are your reactions slow? • Do you suffer from dyslexia?	**EFAs** are split into two main groups – omega-3 and omega-6 fatty acids – known as 'essential' as they must be derived from the diet, since the body cannot manufacture them. They are responsible for hormonal balance, nerve transmission, the acuteness of the senses, maintaining supple skin and regulating fat storage.	Omega-3 EFAs: fish and seafood, sesame, sunflower and pumpkin seeds and their oils; omega-6 EFAs: avocados, pumpkin, sunflower, sesame, linseed and hemp seeds and their oils. 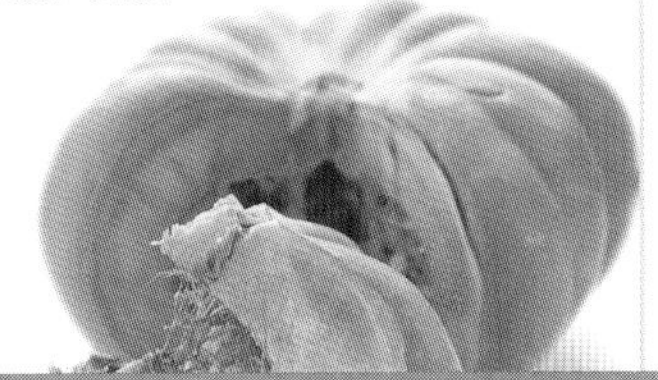

VITAMIN A	FUNCTION	RICHEST SOURCES
• Is your eyesight deteriorating noticeably? • Do you suffer from mouth ulcers? • Do you have cracked lips? • Have you lost your sense of taste? • Do you suffer from frequent colds or infections? • Do you have sinusitis, respiratory problems or excess mucus?	**Vitamin A** is one of the primary antioxidants and is found in two forms – beta-carotene and retinol. Beta-carotene is found in vegetable and fruit sources, whereas retinol comes from animal sources. Vitamin A is vital for eye health and the strength of bones and teeth, as well as for the maintenance of all soft tissue. Most importantly, for sexual health, it is required as an antioxidant for heart and cardiovascular health.	Beta-carotene: dark green leafy vegetables, including kale, Swiss chard, spinach, watercress, broccoli and parsley, and yellow-orange fruit and vegetables, including squash, cantaloupe melon, peaches and tomatoes; retinol: the livers of animals (calves' and pigs' livers), all dairy produce, eggs and oily fish. 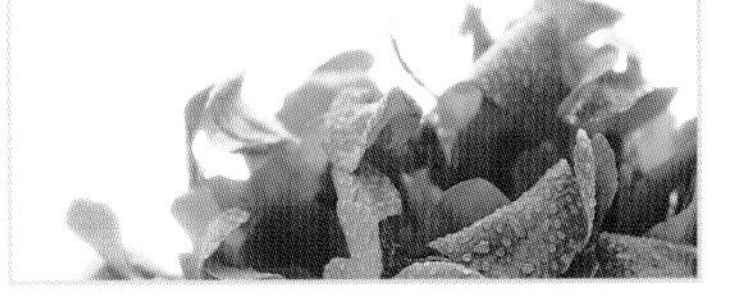

VITAMIN B-COMPLEX including B1, B2, B3, B5, B6, B12, choline	FUNCTION	RICHEST SOURCES
• Are you tired all the time? • Do you suffer from anxiety or nervousness? • Are you sensitive to bright lights? • Is your hair thinning, lank or dry? • Do you experience unexplained muscle twitches? • Do you have dry skin, nails or lips? • Are your eyelids sensitive or red? • Do you suffer from depression? • Do you fail to cope well with stress? • Do you suffer from severe PMS symptoms?	The group of vitamins collectively known as B-complex is the most important one for the production of energy, as well as being vital for protein and carbohydrate digestion. **Vitamin B3** is known as the 'blushing vitamin'. it induces an increase in the flexibility of the capillary walls of the circulatory system, causing them to dilate and allowing more blood to the area (for example, in the penis to stimulate erection). It does this by stimulating histamine (another hormone involved with the immune system), which is required for orgasm. **Vitamin B6** in particular plays a regulatory role in sex-hormone function, and reduces prolactin, which is primarily released to activate lactation when breastfeeding (see p. 62). It also regulates testosterone levels in men, and deficiencies are commonly found in men of viripausal years. **Choline** (which is not strictly a vitamin, but is considered to belong to this group of B vitamins) is the precursor to acetyl-choline – the neurotransmitter required for the transmission of nerve impulses. It is therefore important in boosting energy levels and libido and in creating the 'feel-good' factor.	Wholegrains (especially brown rice) and cereals, pulses, nuts, yeast extracts, meat, fish, eggs, dairy produce, avocados, cream, mushrooms and broccoli. 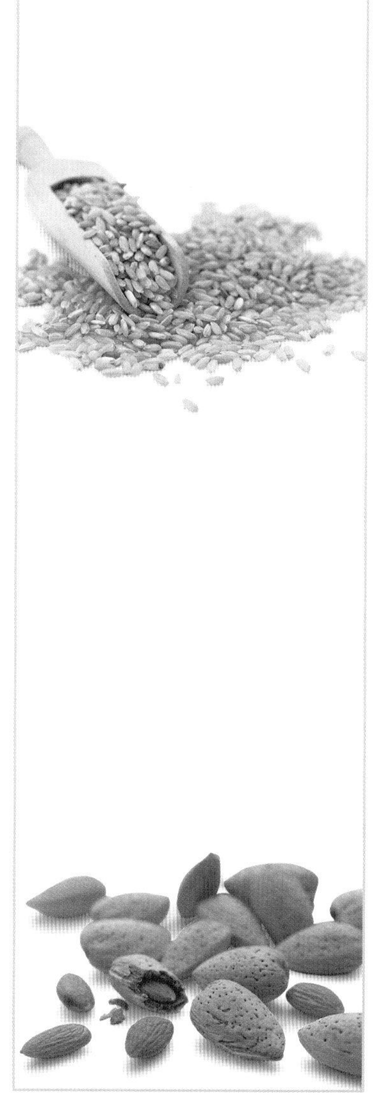

VITAMIN C	FUNCTION	RICHEST SOURCES
• Do you suffer from regular colds or other infections? • Do you have poor skin texture or elasticity? • Do you suffer regularly from bleeding gums? • Do you bruise easily? • Do you have nosebleeds? • Are you slow to heal? • Do you have arterial or venous problems, such as varicose veins? • Do you smoke? • Do you drink alcohol daily?	**Vitamin C** is essential for increasing semen volume, and for ensuring that sperm do not clump together. It also has the capability to boost sex drive and strengthen the sex organs in both men and women.	Raspberries, blackberries, strawberries, citrus fruit, kiwi fruit, mangoes, papayas, figs, potatoes, green peppers, broccoli, beetroot (beet) and sprouted vegetables, such as mung beans and alfalfa sprouts. 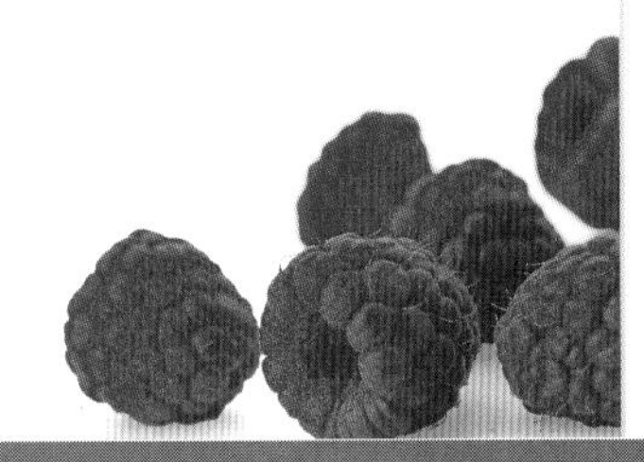

VITAMIN E	FUNCTION	RICHEST SOURCES
• Is your skin dry and inelastic? • Do you have different skin pigmentations over your body? • Are you slow to heal? • Do you suffer from periodic cramping of the legs? • Do you get breathless easily? • Do you have cardiovascular problems such as angina? • Do you have a high cholesterol level? • Do you bruise easily? • Do you suffer from fluid retention? • Do you drink alcohol more than four times a week? • Do you have signs of premature ageing?	**Vitamin E** works together with vitamin C as a potent antioxidant, protecting the heart and cardiovascular system and maintaining the quality of hair, skin and internal tissues. It is probably best known for its skin-healing properties and is often included in skin cosmetics. However, it is the potential internal protective nature of vitamin E that is vital to ensure sexual health and vitality.	All green leafy vegetables, including broccoli, watercress, spinach, parsley, kale and avocados (which have one of the highest vegetable levels of vitamin E), brown rice, nuts and their oils, oatmeal and wheatgerm. 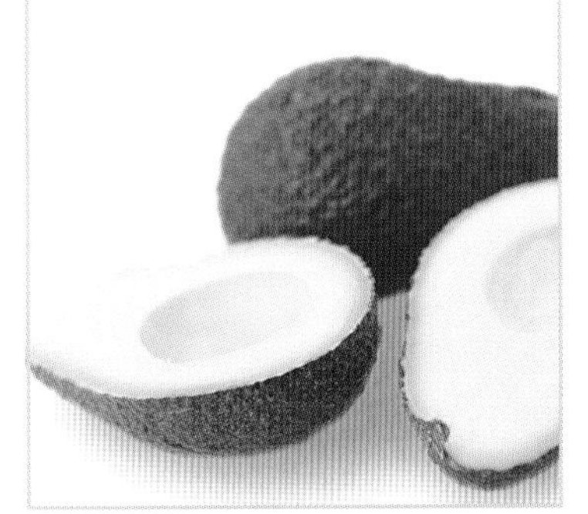

sexy foods

Many foods contain vitamins, minerals and amino acids which can boost your desire and help to remedy sexual problems. From strawberries and oysters to mangoes, pine nuts and asparagus, the following top forty sexy foods reveal the secrets to getting the most out of your bedtime!

Sea bass

♥♥♥♥

This tasty white fish is a good source of omega-3 essential fatty acids which can heighten sexual arousal as well as being vital for sperm formation. Sea bass also contains zinc, magnesium and selenium.

magnesium, omega-3 EFAs, selenium, zinc

Eggs

♥♥♥♥

Eggs provide a rich source of iron, which is found in abundance in the yolk. They also contain zinc, calcium, B vitamins and high-quality protein. All types of eggs (hen, goose, duck, quail, etc.) provide similar nutrients, although perhaps the eggs of battery hens are not considered to be the best choice.

calcium, iron, zinc, B vitamins

Caviar

♥♥♥

These precious fish eggs, long considered a delicacy (partly due to their rarity), contain iron and choline, a member of the B group of vitamins. Magnesium is also found in caviar.

iron, magnesium, B vitamins (especially choline)

Popcorn

♥

Plain popcorn is a rare vegetable source of the amino acid arginine. Amino acids are primarily derived from animal products, so popcorn makes an excellent vegetarian alternative.

arginine

♥ Each heart represents a sexy nutrient.

Rye

♥♥♥♥♥♥

Rich in many minerals that can enhance sexuality, including iron, magnesium and zinc, rye is another good source of energy-enhancing B vitamins, including vitamins B5 and B6, which enhance mood and self-perception. Rye also contains high levels of calcium and vitamin E, as well as phosphorus, magnesium and silicon, which provides cerebral energy.

calcium, iron, magnesium, zinc, vitamins B and E

Spinach

♥♥♥♥♥♥♥

Eaten raw, spinach is one of the few vegetables that contains co-enzyme Q10; it is also one of the most well-known sources of iron. In addition, spinach is a rich source of folic acid, beta-carotene, vitamins B3, B6, vitamin C, calcium and magnesium

beta-carotene, calcium, co-enzyme Q10, iron, magnesium, vitamins B and C

Tofu

♥♥♥♥♥

This low-fat, versatile food contains phyto-oestrogens – substances which mimic the actions of natural oestrogens, which are renowned for harmonizing female hormones. Tofu is widely used in Asian countries, where there is a far lower rate of hormonal complications than in the West. Tofu is also high in iron, calcium, magnesium and vitamin A.

calcium, iron, magnesium, phyto-oestrogens, vitamin A

Pine nuts

♥♥♥♥

All seeds and nuts are prime vegetarian sources of protein, providing the essential building blocks for sexual development. Pine nuts are a rich source of minerals, especially zinc and magnesium, as well as of B vitamins and calcium, all of which are helpful in sustaining energy and creating stamina.

calcium, magnesium, zinc, B vitamins

Strawberries ♥♥♥♥♥♥

This succulent fruit is packed with vitamin C. It also contains iron, which is well absorbed by the body because of the presence of the vitamin C; and beta-carotene, folic acid, vitamin E, calcium and magnesium. Delicious eaten on their own, strawberries also make decorative additions to numerous puddings, as well as an excellent and colourful ingredient in smoothies.

beta-carotene, calcium, iron, magnesium, vitamins C and E

Avocados ♥♥♥♥♥

Avocados contain two vitamins that are vital for overall sexual performance: vitamin B6, and vitamin E. A deficiency of these vitamins is associated with low sex drive and reduced fertility. Avocados are also high in iron, beta-carotene, folic acid and vitamins B3 and B6.

beta-carotene, EFAs, iron, vitamins B and E

Ginger ♥♥♥♥♥♥

As a stimulant, ginger is known to help thin the blood, encouraging increased and prolonged erectile function. It contains beta-carotene, vitamin C, calcium, iron, zinc and magnesium and is one of the oldest-known aphrodisiacs. Ginger can either be used on its own to make a delicious tea or added to a variety of dishes.

beta-carotene, calcium, iron, magnesium, zinc, vitamin C

Mangoes ♥♥

This delicious fruit was once considered a delicacy, but is now commonplace in many supermarkets. It is rich in beta-carotene, which is required for the production of the sex hormones oestrogen and testosterone. Mango is also a good source of vitamin C, which is necessary for ensuring that sperm do not clump together (a known cause of infertility).

beta-carotene, vitamin C

Almonds

♥♥♥♥♥♥♥

These delicious nuts are a rich source of magnesium and of the essential fatty acids that regulate prostaglandins, which are required for the production of sex hormones. In addition, they are high in calcium, zinc, folic acid and vitamins B2, B3 and E. They are therefore an important food in helping to prevent infertility, as well as in increasing libido.

calcium, magnesium, omega-3 and omega-6 EFAs, zinc, vitamins B and E

Prawns (shrimp)

♥♥♥♥♥♥

As shellfish, prawns (shrimp) contain abundant zinc, magnesium, calcium, iodine and selenium. They are also a rich source of an amino acid (protein derivative) known as phenylalanine, which is required for the production of neurotransmitters in the brain that regulate mood and increase sexual appetite.

calcium, iodine, magnesium, phenylalanine, selenium, zinc

Sesame seeds

♥♥♥♥♥♥♥♥

These tiny seeds belie their nutritional wealth. They contain one of the highest sources of the vital trace element selenium, plus ample zinc, which is always an important nutritional element when considering possible causes of infertility. In addition, they are a good source of calcium, iron, magnesium, vitamin E, folic acid and omega-3 and omega-6 EFAs. It is important to grind the seeds briefly in a blender to release their essential minerals, or to use sesame oil in dressings or to finish stir-fries (never heat the oil, as it will damage the delicate essential fatty acids).

calcium, iron, magnesium, omega-3 and omega-6 EFAs, selenium, zinc, vitamin E

Celery

♥♥♥

Known to stimulate the pituitary gland (the primary gland that stimulates all the other glands that produce sex hormones), celery is also rich in selenium. Celery root has long been considered an aphrodisiac, combining beta-carotene, folic acid and vitamin B6 as well, and is frequently eaten for this purpose in the Far East. It is also an excellent digestive, ideal for munching on after a rich or large meal to ensure that your sexual appetite is not lowered!

beta-carotene, selenium, B vitamins

Garlic ♥♥

Although the strong flavour and odour of garlic are not immediately associated with an aphrodisiac, this versatile vegetable is renowned for its many medicinal attributes – not least for increasing circulation and keeping the arteries clear in order to ensure erectile function in middle age and beyond. Interestingly, hardening of the arteries is a frequent cause of impotence in men, so including garlic regularly in your eating plans is advisable. Garlic is also a rich source of calcium and vitamin C.

calcium, vitamin C

Cream ♥♥♥

Eaten in moderation, cream is considered to be an excellent source of calcium; it is rich in the B-complex vitamins and is also a source of arginine. It makes a luxurious addition to fruit puddings and chocolate dishes.

arginine, calcium, B vitamins

Cheese ♥♥♥♥

Likewise part of the dairy family, cheese contains a balance of calcium and magnesium and also contains arginine. High in zinc, cheese may be considered a good second runner (after seafood) for this important mineral.

arginine, calcium, magnesium, zinc

Brown rice ♥♥♥♥♥

While not necessarily considered a food to indulge in for its own sake, brown rice is nonetheless an abundant source of all the B vitamins. It is a good source of zinc, iron, magnesium, chromium, manganese and calcium, all of which are linked to boosting sex drive. Brown rice is excellent for risotto and other mixed dishes, as well as an accompaniment to game and fish dishes.

calcium, iron, magnesium, zinc, B vitamins

Papayas

♥♥♥♥

In the same category of exotic fruit as mango, with the same levels of beta-carotene and vitamin C, the papaya's delicate orange flesh is deliciously enhanced by adding some lime juice. Perhaps lesser known is the value of the dark pips, or seeds, which can be ground in a blender in the same way as linseeds or sesame seeds, to release their rich supply of essential fats, which are required for stimulating sex-hormone production. Papaya is also a good source of calcium and magnesium.

beta-carotene, calcium, magnesium, vitamin C

Onions and leeks

♥♥♥♥

Originating from the same allium family as garlic, onions and leeks have the same potential to increase sexual function in the male. They are also considered to be liver-supporting foods and, as female oestrogen hormones are conjugated in the liver (in the final stage of the process of hormone manufacture), they may well help to balance the hormones in women, particularly in those who suffer from PMS and menopausal symptoms. Both vegetables are rich in calcium and folic acid, and are also a good source of magnesium and beta-carotene.

beta-carotene, calcium, chromium, magnesium

Prunes

♥♥

Known above all for their digestive characteristics, prunes also contain phyto-oestrogens, which help balance the female hormones. They are rich in iron and calcium.

calcium, iron

Figs

♥♥♥

Long considered one of the most erotic fruits, figs were often used in seventeenth- and eighteenth-century Dutch paintings as a symbol of sexuality or fertility. Their high beta-carotene content ensures the regular production of sex hormones and, as a good source of vitamin C, increases libido (see p. 62) and reduces stress (see p. 44). Figs are also a rich source of calcium.

beta-carotene, calcium, vitamin C

Lentils

♥♥♥♥♥

Although not usually associated with increasing sexual appetite, these power-packed pulses should not be overlooked. As a staple part of the Indian diet (dhal is made from puréed lentils, garlic and onions – all of which are considered to have libido-enhancing properties), lentils are rich sources of the B-complex group of vitamins. Additionally, they are a good source of zinc and manganese, both of which have libido-increasing properties, and also contain calcium and magnesium.

calcium, manganese, magnesium, zinc, B vitamins

Mushrooms and truffles

♥♥♥♥♥

As all mushrooms have a high yeast (mould) content, they are an excellent source of the B-complex group of vitamins. In addition they contain calcium, iron, magnesium and zinc. The wide assortment of mushrooms now readily available affords a multitude of uses – either eaten raw in salads or cooked. Truffles have always been considered an aphrodisiac, partly owing to their odour and partly to their rarity. Truffle oil is a cheaper alternative, and may be used in a variety of recipes.

calcium, iron, magnesium, zinc, B vitamins

Dark chocolate

♥♥♥

Women with PMS often crave chocolate prior to their period, not without good reason, for it is abundant in magnesium, which can help to relax menstrual cramps. Chocolate also contains phenylalanine, the amino acid that affects arousal and enhances mood. Enjoy it (occasionally), and favour the darkest chocolate you can find, but keep it as a treat.

magnesium, phenylalanine, potassium

Tuna

♥♥♥♥

Rich in zinc, selenium, vitamins B12 and B3, protein and omega-3 essential fatty acids, tuna is often regarded as the king of the sexual foods (after oysters). It increases sperm production and raises the libido and stamina. Eaten fresh or tinned, this delicious fish should be a regular part of any man or woman's eating plan.

omega-3 EFAs, selenium, zinc, B vitamins

Asparagus

♥♥♥

Full of nutrients, including folic acid, beta-carotene, vitamin C, this vegetable has many health-giving properties and is considered to be one of the most supportive foods for the liver. As both oestrogens and testosterone are conjugated in the liver, asparagus can help to regulate hormonal imbalances (see p. 42) and increase sexual performance.

beta-carotene, vitamins B and C

Tomatoes

♥♥♥♥♥♥

One of the richest sources of beta-carotene (the precursor of vitamin A, which is converted on the wall of the intestine), a tomato is in fact a fruit, not a vegetable. Vitamin A is essential for the production of male and female sex hormones and for promoting fertility. As an anti-oxidant, beta-carotene promotes heart health.

beta-carotene, calcium, magnesium, vitamins A, B and C

Bananas

♥♥♥♥

The flesh of the banana closest to its skin contains an alkaloid called bufotenine, which affects the balance of neurotransmitters in the brain, to elevate mood and increase self-confidence. As lowered libido (see pp.54 and 59) is often associated with psychological well-being, bananas should be included regularly in the eating plan of anyone who suffers from low self-esteem. They are also rich in beta-carotene and vitamin C.

beta-carotene, magnesium, tryptophan, vitamin C

Blackberries and raspberries

♥♥♥♥♥

Two of the richest sources of vitamin C, these dark fruit are important ingredients on the Sexy Shopping List (see p.36). They are also a good source of vitamin E, which is required for increasing sex drive and maintaining a soft, supple skin. In addition, they are both an excellent source of calcium, magnesium and beta-carotene.

beta-carotene, calcium, magnesium, vitamins C and E

Beetroot (beet)

♥♥♥♥♥

As well as being supportive to the liver, where sexual hormones are conjugated, beetroot (beet) is a rich source of iron, calcium and potassium, all of which are required for healthy circulation. In addition it contains abundant beta-carotene and vitamin C, both of which support and protect the sexual organs.

beta-carotene, calcium, iron, potassium, vitamin C

Pumpkins

♥♥♥♥♥♥♥

Pumpkin's crunchy seeds have recently attracted much attention for their protective properties for prostate health (see p. 56). These seeds are also a great source of calcium, iron, magnesium, zinc and B vitamins. In addition, they are a rich source of omega-3 and omega-6 essential fatty acids, which are required for the production of sex hormones (testosterone in the male). Essential fats are also anti-inflammatory, hence their role in preventing the development of an enlarged prostate. Eaten raw or lightly toasted in olive oil and soy sauce, pumpkin is also delicious added to salads and soups on a frequent basis.

calcium, iron, magnesium, omega-3 and omega-6 EFAs, zinc, B vitamins

Broccoli

♥♥♥♥

Now considered to be one of the most important green vegetable for its myriad health-giving properties (including its role in cancer protection), broccoli also has its place in enhancing sexual function. It is a rich source of iron, B vitamins and vitamins A and C – the last two being primary antioxidants.

iron, vitamins A, B and C

Watercress

♥♥♥♥♥

This slightly sour salad leaf is an abundant source of iron (see p. 18), as well as potassium, both of which are vital for regulating the heart and circulation. It also contains calcium, beta-carotene, magnesium and vitamin C. Usually eaten raw, watercress is known for its blood-cleansing properties, making it a valuable food for any man with erectile dysfunction (see p. 52) owing to cardiovascular problems.

beta-carotene, calcium, iron, magnesium, vitamin C

♥ **Each heart represents a sexy nutrient.**

Herbs and spices

Aside from enhancing flavour, herbs and spices can have many effects on sexual function. Use them raw or cook them, and in the case of tarragon and basil, add a few leaves to a bottle of olive oil for a delicious and versatile dressing.

Saffron

special properties

These tiny topaz-coloured strands (the dried stigmas of the crocus plant) are the world's most expensive spice. They have long been considered in India to have sexually stimulating effects that justify their considerable expense. Only saffron from the Asian saffron crocus (**Crocus sativus**), which is harvested at certain times of the year, has a particular potency for the male libido.

sexually stimulating

Tarragon

special properties

Tarragon's strong flavour indicates its stimulatory effects on the heart and liver. This herb is considered to be a blood cleanser and tonifier, increasing circulation and maintaining arterial health. As a support to the liver, it enhances the conjugation of sex hormones (oestrogen and testosterone).

stimulating, cleansing, increases circulation

Nutmeg

special properties

In the seventeenth century the English and Dutch fought to control the nutmeg trade from the Spice Islands and nutmeg was considered to have aphrodisiac properties. In normal use it is reputed to be a sexual stimulant. Large doses can be toxic.

sexually stimulating

Basil

special properties

Possibly the freshest-tasting herb, basil has both calming and anti-stress properties (see p. 44), as well as being considered a sexual stimulant. It is used as the main ingredient in pesto or pistou (see p. 138), together with pine nuts and garlic – a combination that cannot fail to raise excitement levels.

calming, anti-stress, sexually stimulating

sexy weekend

To prepare for this indulgent weekend, think of spoiling yourselves in every way. While you may wish to adhere to the general principles of blood-sugar management (see p. 40) to ensure prolonged stamina, you also want to ensure sufficient rest and relaxation, which are equally important. Planning ahead is therefore essential (see the shopping list on p.36) – you don't want to find that you have forgotten the magic ingredient at the wrong moment.

Note: if you are not fond of fish, try the **Ginger and Pineapple Chicken** recipe instead (see p. 117) – ginger is a wonderful stimulant for all kinds of activities.

Optional pudding: if you have not eaten enough by this stage, try the **Banana Custard** recipe (see p. 122) for a sinful, yet beneficial pudding. This can be prepared at the time or earlier in the day.

FOOD PLAN

FRIDAY NIGHT

Start the weekend with total indulgence: six fresh oysters each, with a wedge of fresh lemon and black pepper – nothing more is needed. Follow this with **Fennel, Apple and Almond Salad** (see p. 114), with a simple olive oil and lemon dressing, or a similar light salad. Serve with a glass of champagne for maximum benefit!

SATURDAY

Breakfast/brunch

Eggs are important for energy and stamina, and our recipe for **Baked Eggs with Spinach** (see p. 111) is the perfect breakfast or light lunch (assuming you haven't risen too early!). Enjoy this dish with some toasted rye bread or pumpernickel for maximum energy and healthy all-round nutrition.

Mid-afternoon snack

For the perfect snack that won't ruin your appetite for the evening, choose a light but power-packed food, such as avocado dip with blue corn chips, which will ensure that your moods are kept balanced and your energy levels restored. See our **Green Velvet recipe** (p. 124) for this easy snack, which can be prepared in a minute.

Dinner

Take time preparing dinner together, and enjoy the shared experience that cooking has to offer. Start with tiny quails' eggs, which only need boiling for one minute, then allow them to stand for a further minute before running them under cold water and removing the shells. Serve on a bed of watercress or rocket with your favourite dressing (see p. 112 for an alternative idea of **Watercress, Orange and Sesame-Seed Salad**). For your main course, see the recipe for **Grilled Tuna with Mint and Parsley Salsa** (p. 118) – you may wish to use limes instead of lemons, for a change in flavour. Serve with steamed broccoli and snowpeas to include fibre and added vitamins.

Abstain from coffee, which will simply interfere with your sleep later in the night. Instead, enjoy a cup of green tea (which has immune-building properties and less than half the caffeine of regular tea) or ginger and lemon tea (which follows the flavours of the rest of the meal, to give you a clean finish to your dinner).

SUNDAY

Breakfast

For an easy-to-prepare breakfast in a glass, see the recipe for **Raspberry and Mango Smoothie** (p. 110), which is literally a meal-in-a-minute, and absolutely delicious. If this just whets your appetite for more, or you find yourselves really hungry, follow with **Creamy Porridge with Prunes** (see p. 111).

Lunch

Rather than preparing a traditional heavy Sunday lunch, why not have a lighter dish, such as **Broad Bean, Pea and Asparagus Risotto** (see p. 121), which is simple to cook and is a good source of vegetable protein and fibre, ensuring that you don't reach the end of your wonderful weekend feeling heavy and over-full.

Evening meal

If you still feel hungry in the evening, have a plate of smoked salmon and fresh lemon with the remainder of the rye or pumpernickel bread for a well-balanced light meal, and top off with a half-bottle of dry white wine, such as Sancerre or Chardonnay. Retire early!

SHOPPING LIST

You need to buy enough fresh produce to see you through until breakfast on Monday, so that you do not have to interrupt your lazy weekend with food shopping. If the suggested produce is out of season, choose other seasonal fruits or vegetables – the important factor here is variety and freshness. The quantities given below are for two people.

You will also need to add the ingredients for some of the following recipes to your shopping list. Carefully read through the food plan (see p.35) and decide which of the recipes you will need ingredients for.

Fennel, Apple and Almond Salad (see p.114)
Baked Eggs with Spinach (see p.111)
Green Velvet (see p. 124)
Watercress, Orange and Sesame Seed Salad (see p.112) [an alternative to the bunch of watercress or rocket (arugula)]
Grilled Tuna with Mint and Parsley Salsa (see p.118) or Ginger and Pineapple Chicken (see p.117)
Banana Custard (see p.122) [optional]
Raspberry and Mango Smoothie (p.110)
Creamy Porridge with Prunes (see p.111) [optional]
Broad Bean, Pea and Asparagus Risotto (see p.121)

12 fresh oysters
2 lemons
loaf of rye bread or pumpernickel
blue or yellow corn chips
12 quails' eggs
bunch of watercress or rocket (arugula)
1 head of broccoli
8oz/250g snowpeas or mangetout
8oz/250g smoked salmon
Japanese green tea or herbal tea of your choice
small piece of fresh root ginger (for tea)
bottle of good champagne
half bottle of dry white wine

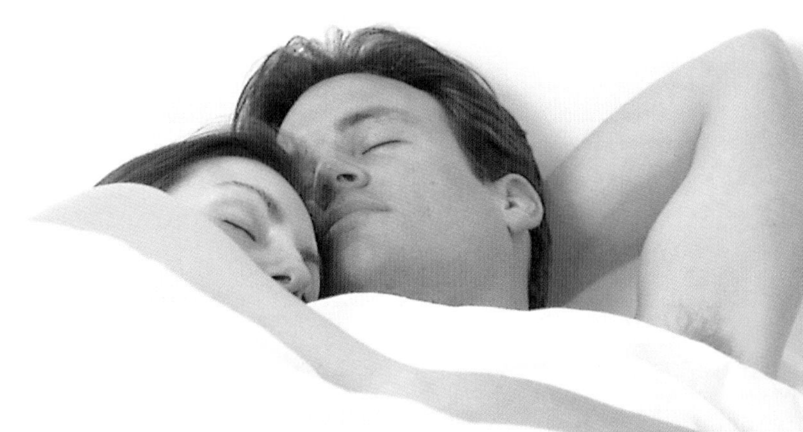

ESSENTIAL TIPS

1 Remember to drink plenty of water throughout the day to maintain maximum hydration – sex is very dehydrating.
2 Ensure that you have no interruptions – switch on the answering machine.
3 Discourage friends and family from visiting.
4 Make sure that the household chores are done before the weekend.
5 Invest in some new underwear (preferably not your usual, day-to-day brand).
6 Scented candles for the bedroom and bathroom add sensuality and set the mood.

Drinks

Have some fine wine or champagne, but do not drink alcohol to excess.
Drink plenty of water, flavoured with fresh cucumber or mint leaves for added freshness.
Ginseng tea is beneficial and tea made with fresh root ginger is stimulating.

Essential oils

Essential oils can be used in various different ways to stimulate the body and enhance the senses – in the bath, in a vaporizer or by putting just a few drops of neat oil on your shirt collar. Never use essential oils neat on the skin, as they must be combined with a base oil such as almond. Different herbs have different qualities, but the following are arousing in one way or another:

Ylang-ylang – stimulating and invigorating
Sandalwood – rich and sensual
Orange blossom – fragrant and uplifting
Geranium – warming and long-lasting
Allspice berry – spicy and enhances the senses
Caraway – enhances the circulation

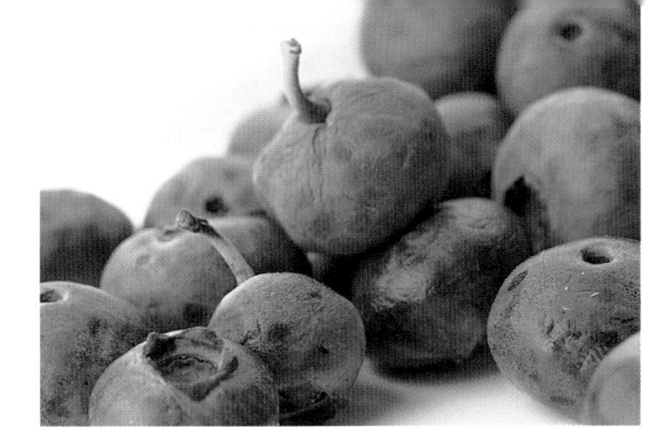

what

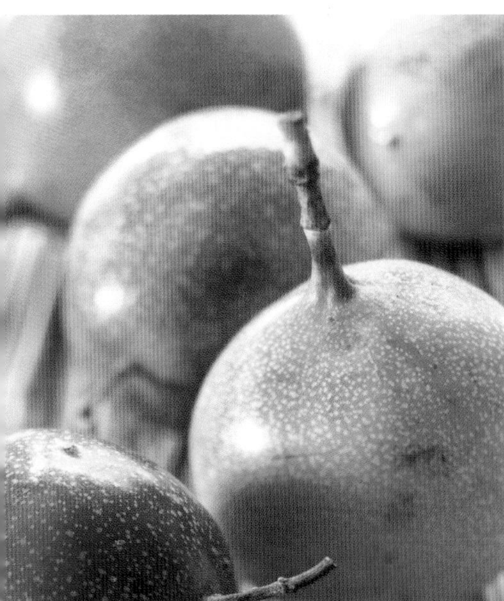

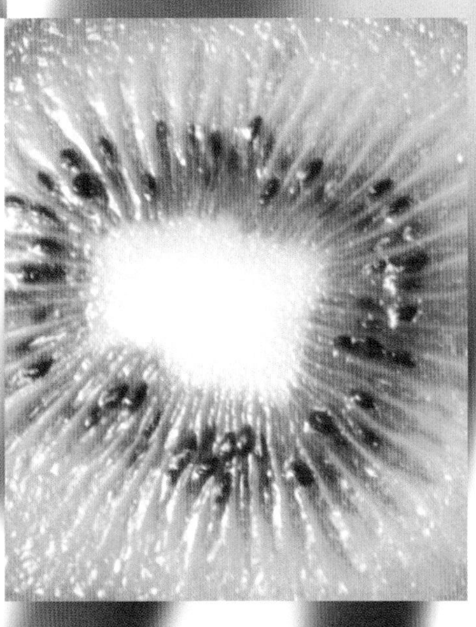

can go wrong?

factors which control your sex drive and libido

Inevitably, there are factors in our everyday lives that can have a profound effect on our sex drive and libido. These include hormone imbalances, stress, specific nutritional deficiences and general poor eating habits, as well as over use of processed foods and stimulants.

So if we want to boost our libido and remedy any sexual problems, we need to ensure that our metabolic hormones are balanced. Brain neurotransmitters (chemicals that conduct messages from one nerve ending to another), such as serotonin, dopamine and acetylcholine, also have a stimulatory or inhibitory effect on our levels of desire, stimulation and arousal. When our levels of these chemicals are low or out of balance, this impacts on our libido.

Psychological stimuli – sight and imagination – play an active role in our levels of reaction as well, as do the physical stimuli of taste, touch and smell. The brain processes every aspect of sexual pleasure, so our senses and emotions are vital factors in our sex drive.

Virtually the entire body is thus involved in some way in the process of arousal, desire and the act of sex. While it is important to create the right environment for stimulating attraction in the first place, there is nothing as potent for the body as an optimum diet to ensure vitality, energy, a good sense of self-esteem and confidence. It is therefore useful to know which specific foods have positive effects on boosting libido in both men and women. The following pages look at some of the problems – physical and emotional, male and female – that can affect your sex drive, and then at some libido-boosters (see p. 6) that can help to remedy the situation, in both men and women.

problems

Any one of the following health conditions can affect sexual function yet it is possible to counteract these problems with everyday foods. If the questionnaire on pages 12 to 15 highlighted any areas that require attention, then use this section to find nutritional solutions.

blood-sugar imbalances

Imbalances in blood-sugar levels can affect both sexual desire and performance. If you are feeling fatigued, with highs and lows of energy throughout the day, then this is likely to have a profound effect on your self-perception and on your general interest in sex. Most of us are familiar with the peaks and troughs that we feel every day. Lowered blood-sugar levels are responsible for the hunger and fatigue that many people experience mid-afternoon, yet these changes actually happen throughout the day, albeit in a less pronounced fashion.

Much of the food that we eat is converted by a series of biochemical processes into glucose, which is the ideal source of fuel for the body. Glucose circulates in the blood and tissues to provide an energy source for every single cell, and blood-sugar levels are tightly controlled through the action of various hormones. As food is digested and assimilated, glucose levels in the blood rise, triggering the release of insulin from the pancreas. Insulin is essentially a storage hormone that facilitates the entry of glucose into the cells through a series of receptors on their surface. When stimulated, these receptors open channels to allow glucose to flow into the cell.

BALANCING PRINCIPLES

In order to create consistent energy, these guidelines should be followed:

1. Always combine protein, carbohydrates and fibre at every meal and snack.
2. Eat small but frequent meals, perhaps four or five times daily.
3. Snack between meals, remembering to combine the various food groups.
4. Avoid sweet foods.
5. Reduce your stimulant intake (including coffee, tea and carbonated drinks).
6. Avoid processed food and eat a diet that is rich in fresh wholefoods.

Foods are converted into glucose at differing speeds. For example, a simple sugar (such as honey) is converted into energy almost instantly, whereas a complex carbohydrate (such as brown rice) takes longer to be broken down into glucose. If a meal comprises only simple carbohydrates, then glucose levels rise quickly, providing instant energy, but also triggering the release of insulin, which can precipitate the increase of fat storage. Blood-sugar levels that rise quickly will fall at the same speed, and we experience this as highs and lows in our energy levels, mood and ability to concentrate.

Proteins are more difficult to digest, therefore releasing glucose into the blood at a slower rate. In turn, this ensures that the demand for insulin production is also slower and more consistent, providing a longer period of sustained energy and alleviating fluctuations in energy levels and mood.

Using food to balance blood-sugar levels

By choosing certain foods you can help avoid the marked high and lows. As a general rule, carbohydrates release their sugars quickly (and simple carbohydrates do so more quickly than those that are considered complex), whilst proteins do so at a far slower rate. Fibre and fats further slow down the release of sugars and should be eaten at every meal. The key is to graze – or eat 'little and often' – to ensure that your energy levels remain consistent. Eating two or three large meals a day places a burden on the digestive system, as a result of which the pancreatic demand for insulin production is higher. Eating a smaller meal every three to four hours is preferable.

Insulin resistance

We will see (p. 44) how stress can raise blood-sugar levels through the action of adrenaline, and we have already seen how the action of insulin facilitates the entry of glucose into the body's cells. Over time cells may fail to recognize the presence of insulin, and the relevant channels will not open to accept the glucose molecules. Blood-sugar levels remain high, causing the pancreas to release more insulin. The cycle continues until the cells finally open to accept glucose, causing sugar levels in the blood to tumble and we experience this as fatigue.

Excessive insulin production may be pro-inflammatory, and is often found to be involved in inflammatory conditions such as irritable bowel syndrome, rheumatoid arthritis and eczema. It is also the major factor in type II diabetes. When this condition remains chronic for an extended period it may result in late-onset diabetes, requiring medicated insulin supplementation, so it makes sense to keep a close eye on your blood-sugar levels.

PERFECT BSBS (BLOOD-SUGAR BALANCE SNACKS)

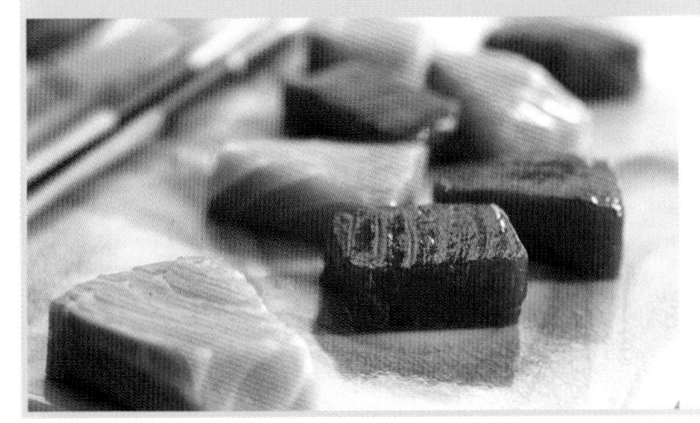

- Ryvita and cottage cheese with a watercress topping
- Oat cakes, hummus and alfalfa sprouts
- Apple and a chunk of Cheddar
- Sardines on toast with sliced tomato
- Sushi box – fish or vegetarian
- Cup of chicken and vegetable soup

hormonal imbalances

There are many causes of hormonal imbalances, some of which result from external stimuli and others from the complex interaction of the body's organ functions. The body is in a state of constant change and flux, trying to reach a metabolic balance, a state known as 'homeostasis'. In order to achieve this, the endocrine glands (which secrete hormones into the bloodstream) will compensate for hormone-level fluctuations by stimulating other hormones into production.

For example, if you have been under long-term stress due to work or other pressures, or are suffering from an illness such as a heart condition or high blood pressure, the adrenal glands will overwork to maintain increased heart-muscle contraction (activated by the adrenals releasing both adrenaline and cortisol). Over a period of time the adrenal glands become fatigued through overuse and require rest and recovery. This is achieved by lowering the rate of metabolism, forcing you to slow down and sleep longer hours. The body's metabolic rate is controlled by the thyroid gland, which is found at the base of the throat, just behind the Adam's apple area. Typical signs of lowered thyroid function (see p. 51) include gradual, unexplained weight gain, forgetfulness, fatigue, feeling tearful for no apparent reason and low-grade depression.

Toxins

An ever-increasing number of external factors can have a profound effect on the body's hormonal balance. Many of these derive from the huge array of chemicals that are found in our environment on a daily basis. It is estimated that the average Western person is exposed to approximately 3,000 different chemicals every year, placing a huge demand on the body to detoxify and maintain health.

These chemicals are all around us, in the water that we drink and the air that we breathe, and even before birth we are exposed on a daily basis to these pollutants, many of which can never be broken down and neutralized. Depending on the strength of our immune system, such exposure places an immediate or long-term stress on the body's state of balance.

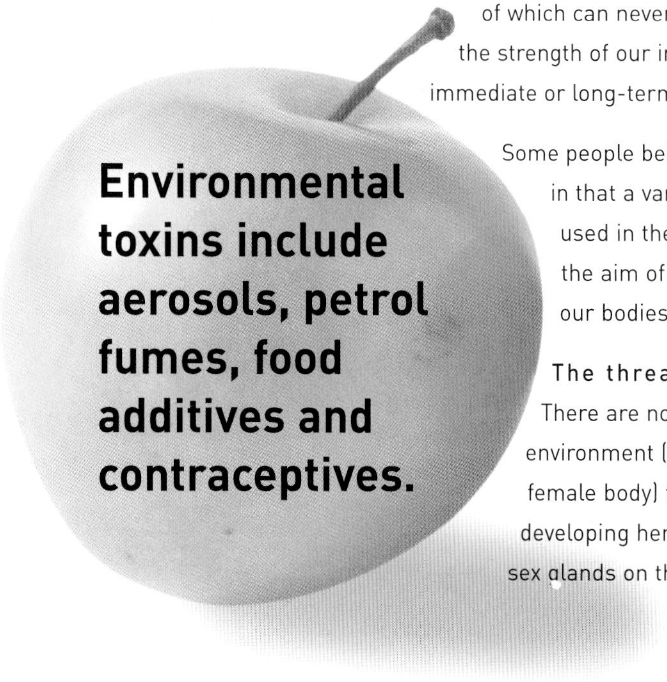

Environmental toxins include aerosols, petrol fumes, food additives and contraceptives.

Some people believe that non-organic food is potentially harmful, in that a variety of herbicides, pesticides and antibiotics is used in the growing, rearing or production of the food (with the aim of increasing its shelf-life) – but at what price to our bodies?

The threat to fertility

There are now so many oestrogen-like compounds in our environment (oestrogens being the major sex hormone in the female body) that some species of sea- and freshwater fish are developing hermaphrodite sex glands (both male and female sex glands on the same animal).

Danish research has also disclosed the alarming fact that, apart from in Sweden (where soil levels of selenium are unusually high – selenium being required for testicular health), the rate of male fertility in the rest of the Western world halved from 1938 to 1992. Despite the worldwide danger of overpopulation, this reduction in male fertility is seen by many as a real threat to the continuation of the human race. It is in part caused by the oestrogen-like compounds, and although oestrogen is not a major hormone in the male sex glands, it is found there in small amounts. Increased exposure to industrial and household pollutants, animal-hormone stimulation and household plastics has tipped our delicate hormonal balance, with potentially devastating repercussions.

Nutritional self-protection

Drinking filtered or bottled water is possibly the most protective measure – recycled water still carries trace amounts of xeno-oestrogens ('xeno' meaning 'false'), bleaches and purifiers, which add to the total toxic load that the body has to deal with on a daily basis. This can slow down liver efficiency, reducing the likelihood of complete detoxification.

Organic animal produce is perhaps a more important consideration than organic fruit and vegetables, as most non-organic cattle raised for dairy production or meat are fed with low-grade antibiotics to prevent infection, and with hormones to increase their bulk or milk flow. Poultry is treated in the same way – an organic chicken breast is half the size of its non-organic counterpart, and this is explained partly by the hormones that are used to bulk up the non-organic variety. The specific influences that long-term intake of additional hormones have on us cannot yet be quantified, but it is certainly not what Nature intended.

PROTECTIVE NUTRIENTS

The liver has to detoxify all potentially harmful chemicals that enter the body. It is also the site of hormone regulation and conversion. Any kind of overload is therefore bound to affect the liver's overall function, and particularly its detoxification processes. The nutrients required to support the liver are specifically vitamin A (see p.21), the B-complex vitamins (see p. 22), including biotin and folic acid, vitamin C (see p.23) and the minerals zinc (see p.18), magnesium (see p.19) and manganese. The majority of these essential nutrients can be supplied by a regular intake of seafood, wholegrains and a variety of green leafy vegetables, rich red berry fruit and a selection of seeds, such as pumpkin, sesame and sunflower.

the stress factor

Stress can reduce sexual desire and function, but how does this happen? We have an inbuilt response to stress, which was designed to protect the body for short periods of time. However, stress – from work, relationships or financial pressures, for example – is rarely a short-term occurrence; modern stresses can occur almost constantly and be so familiar that we can exist in a semi-stressed state without truly acknowledging it.

The body's response

When the body senses danger, or is under pressure in any way, the 'flight or fight' response is triggered. This sets off a series of biochemical changes designed to support the body until the danger in question has passed. Energy is diverted away from the digestive system to provide reserves for the muscles. This reduces the absorption rate of nutrients from food, many of which are essential for sexual function and desire.

Finding ways of leaving stresses outside the bedroom can in turn work to alleviate the causes of stress.

Another equally important influence is the action of the hormone adrenaline. At times of stress, the adrenal glands near the kidneys produce adrenaline, which has many different effects, one of which is to force the release of glucose that is stored in the muscles and liver in the form of glycogen. This raises blood-sugar levels, providing a source of short-term energy. However, as stresses are now being experienced more frequently than our bodies were designed to cope with, this can lead to marked fluctuations in blood-sugar levels (see p. 40). Such fluctuations contribute to feelings of fatigue, listlessness and apathy.

Stress, sex and sleep

It is interesting to note that at times of stress the blood thickens, as the body attempts to reduce blood loss in case of an injury. Thickened blood is a major cause of headaches, which in themselves have become a regular excuse for avoiding sexual relations. Quite apart from the nutritional deficiencies that stress can exacerbate, being mentally preoccupied with problems obviously influences the likelihood of sexual desire. Finding ways of leaving stresses outside the bedroom can in turn work to alleviate the causes of stress.

The fact that sleep plays such an important role in libido is one of the reasons why we have combined these two major topics in one book, for they are dependent on each other – sex and sleep. Remember, too, that sex is a great stress reliever. If you can entice your partner to engage in sexual activity when he or she has been suffering from stress-related insomnia, you will be doing them a huge favour. Research has shown that the quality of sleep is enhanced by sex, as it relaxes the body and mind. Finding the balance between when it is right and when it is not is up to the individual.

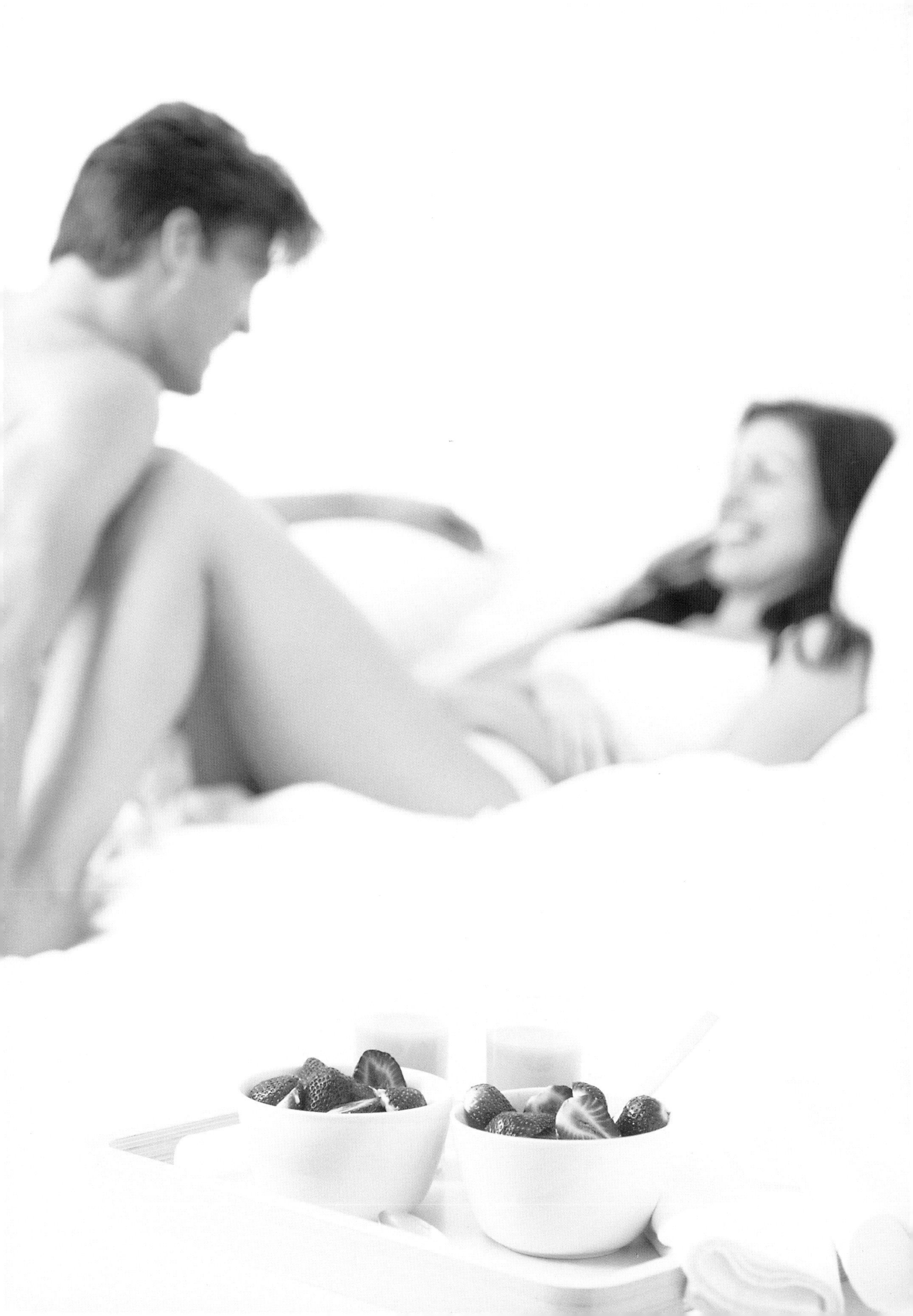

ALCOHOL AND DRUGS

The use of alcohol and recreational drugs is often mistakenly thought to increase sex drive, libido and/or sexual performance. However, as shown below, they invariably interfere with our sexuality, as the senses of stimulation, smell and sight become disrupted in some way. Excessive amounts of alcohol or drugs are often taken to 'reduce inhibition', although in reality they can reduce a man's ability to maintain an erection or the ability of either sex to reach orgasm.

ALCOHOL

While small or moderate amounts of alcohol may act as an aphrodisiac by making people more tactile and less inhibited, the longer-term effects are inevitably detrimental to sexuality in all areas. Alcohol is detoxified by the liver, where the male and female hormones are all conjugated. Regular or excessive intake of alcohol significantly lowers testosterone levels in males, leading to a reduction in the size of the testicles and lowered sperm production, as well as loss of ability to maintain an erection. In women it interferes with oestrogen production, lowering sex drive and reducing vaginal secretions and fertility.

CANNABIS

Short-term use of cannabis reduces inhibition and can stimulate heightened senses. However, long-term or regular use has been shown, in numerous trials, to significantly lower sperm count and motility (the speed and agility of the sperm) and to reduce overall libido by lowering testosterone production.

ECSTASY

Frequently taken as the 'sexy drug' (although it was originally developed as the 'truth drug' for criminal and psychological testing), ecstasy appears to heighten the senses of smell and touch. It is very dehydrating to the body, though, and often leads to a reduction of vaginal fluids, making sexual activity uncomfortable for women. In the long term or with frequent use, ecstasy has been found to damage the thyroid gland, which regulates our metabolic rate and energy production.

COCAINE

This drug has a detrimental effect on erectile function, both during and after use. Known to increase libido in the first instance by elevating blood pressure, cocaine carries a risk of inducing heart attacks and angina. It can also interfere with sperm production and development, as well as disrupting the hormonal balance throughout the body.

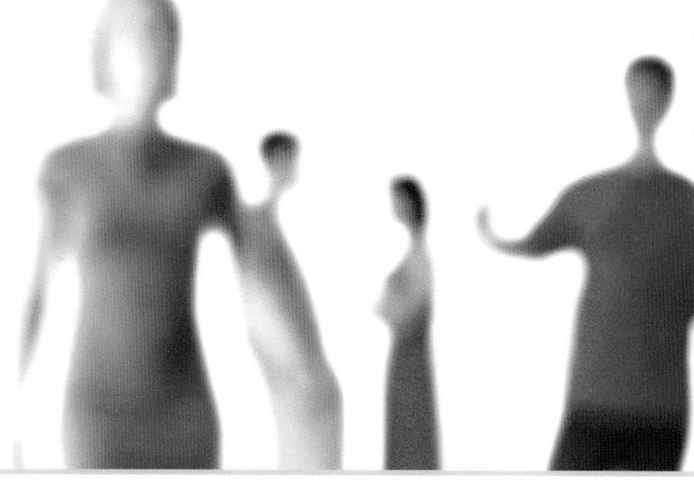

STRESS-BUSTERS

We have seen how stress reduces the body's digestive capabilities and the absorption of virtually all nutrients. Excessive or repetitive stress depletes the body of three main nutrients, which are required specifically (but not solely) for the support of the adrenal glands. Deficiencies of any – or all – of these nutrients lead to further stress, as the adrenals rapidly become exhausted without them.

VITAMIN C

DEFICIENCY SYMPTOMS
mouth ulcers, colds, chapped lips, dry skin

FOUND IN
sweet peppers, broccoli, red berry fruit, kiwi fruit, potatoes, watermelons

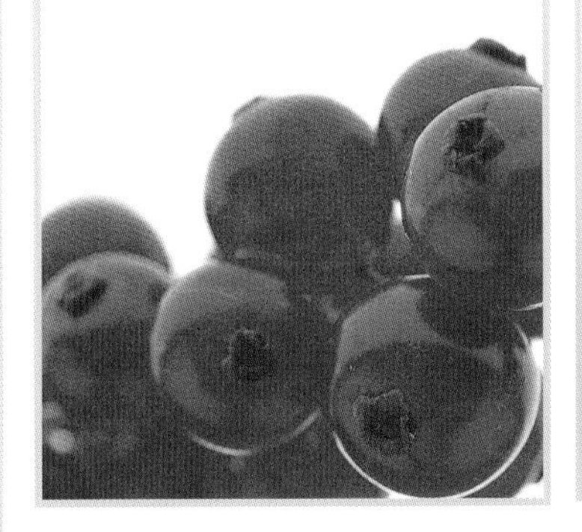

VITAMIN B3

DEFICIENCY SYMPTOMS
depression, lethargy, irritability

FOUND IN
green leafy vegetables, rice, peanuts, wheatgerm

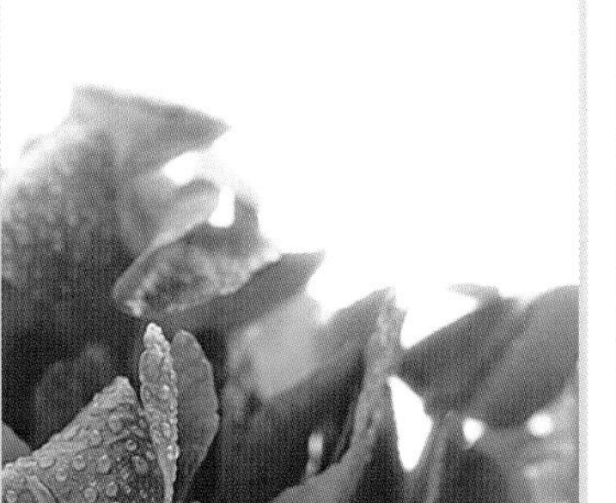

MAGNESIUM

DEFICIENCY SYMPTOMS
muscle twitches, insomnia, irritability, lack of focus

FOUND IN
wholegrains, nuts, green vegetables, all fruit

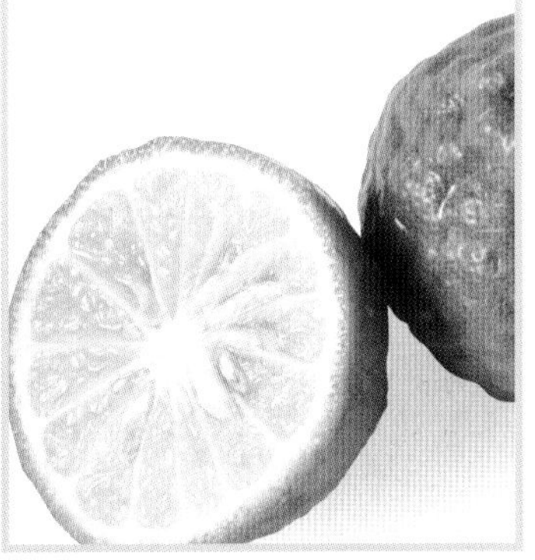

depression

Depression comes in many forms. There is clinical depression, bipolar disorder (more commonly known as manic depression), unipolar depression, seasonal affective disorder (SAD) and dysthymia, which is by far the most prevalent.

Dysthymia comprises one or repeated bouts of depression, which are not debilitating in the extreme, but are responsible for feelings of sadness, anxiety, feeling 'down' or 'blue'. These are very common symptoms and are sometimes event-linked, sometimes seasonal, or may occur for no apparent reason. People with this type of depression are often not treated with medication, as their symptoms are not severe, but obviously they have an effect on one's quality of life. One of the symptoms of depression is a change in appetite – usually a loss of interest in food – which can further exacerbate any nutritional deficiencies that may be involved.

SYMPTOMS

The symptoms of depression are varied, but include:
- Changes in eating habits (usually either loss of appetite or cravings)
- Fatigue
- Disinterest in hobbies and usual pastimes
- Irritability
- Feelings of emptiness
- Insomnia or interrupted sleep patterns, such as early waking

Sex and depression

One of the most common symptoms of all types of depression is the loss of sexual desire. One study in the US found that approximately 33 per cent of all people reported a loss of sexual desire over a given year, but the figure was far higher for those suffering from depression, at over 70 per cent, highlighting the association between libido and mood. While this figure relates to those people who were not on medication, there is also a link between some types of common medication and loss of sexual desire. Anti-depressants may work well in alleviating depression, but perversely loss of sexual desire or ability is an acknowledged side-effect of many drugs.

In men, inability to achieve an erection (see p. 52) or orgasm is common, while in women loss of libido (see p. 59) and altered orgasm are more frequent occurrences. The issue is further complicated by the fact that one or two anti-depressants that are less commonly prescribed these days are thought to increase the desire for sex, yet can cause priapism (persistent and painful erection) in extreme cases.

Despite these potential side-effects and anomalies, what you eat can play a profound role in how you feel, and many clients have felt a 'lifting' of some of the symptoms of depression when following a better diet. This in turn can affect your libido and desire. As depression affects self-perception, any alleviation of the condition will in turn improve this, making you feel more sexual. However, if you are suffering from continued feelings of depression, then it is always wise to consult your health professional.

Mood foods

While we are not suggesting that eating any one food will ease depression, there are interesting links between the food that we turn to for comfort and some of the causes of depression.

The mechanism for boosting neurotransmitters in the brain involves tryptophan, an amino acid that is also responsible for inducing sleep (see p. 106). When we eat carbohydrates (either simple or complex), they suppress the group of amino acids that are vying with one another to cross the blood-brain barrier. Only tryptophan remains relatively unaffected, allowing it to pass unhindered into the brain, where it acts as a precursor to serotonin – and it is serotonin levels that have a direct correlation to the incidence of depression.

There is little doubt that eating a sugary treat, such as a tub of your favourite ice cream, can lift your spirits, but it is not just the 'guilty pleasure' that can help boost your mood. Serotonin levels are indeed increased by carbohydrates, and the higher the sugar levels, the quicker this mechanism is thought to work. However, the link between serotonin and testosterone (see p. 54) is likely to mean that any foods that raise serotonin levels can potentially reduce testosterone levels via the dopamine pathway.

Dopamine acts as a neurotransmitter and requires proteins for its synthesis. This highlights the requirement for a variety of foods – some from each food group, to help maintain mood and fight off depression.

FEEL-BRIGHT NUTRIENTS

The B group of vitamins (see p. 22) is of particular importance in lifting mood – especially B6, which is involved in the synthesis of serotonin, and B9 (folic acid) and B12, which are required for the synthesis of dopamine. Vitamin B3 levels have been found to be low in those suffering from depression, and increasing levels of this water-soluble nutrient is believed to combat it.

The minerals zinc (see p. 18) and magnesium (see p. 19) are also implicated in effectively managing depression. Magnesium is required for dopamine production, and although zinc is not involved as directly in neurotransmitter production, low levels are associated with depression. It is believed that post-partum depression is linked to zinc levels, as much of the mother's zinc passes through the placenta to the child in the days immediately before labour. Zinc is known as the 'growth' mineral as it is responsible in no small way for enhancing this activity. The low zinc levels in mothers of newborns are further highlighted by the concentration of zinc in colostrum (fore-milk), the yellowish liquid that precedes milk on each breastfeeding occasion.

Selenium (see p. 20) has also been found to be lacking in the blood plasma of people suffering from depression. Its antioxidant properties protect against damaging neuro-toxins, such as mercury, which is found in amalgam fillings in teeth.

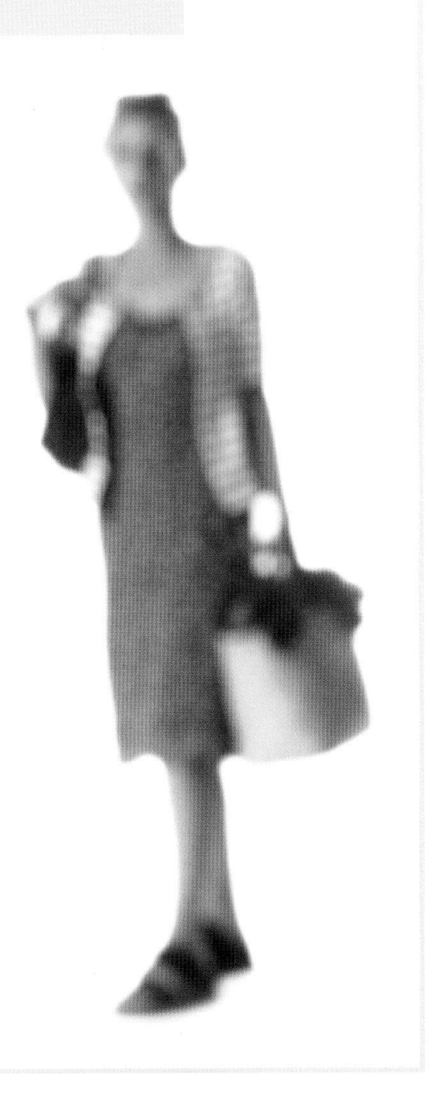

Depression and food allergies

Food allergies have become more widespread in recent years. Much has been made in the press of this increase, but on the whole most food allergies are more likely to be food 'intolerances'.

A food allergy involves a swift response by the immune system, but food intolerances are more subtle and their effects are usually cumulative. In theory, we can be intolerant to any food, yet the most common cause is wheat and wheat flour. These are used in a huge variety of foods, from obvious sources such as bread and pasta to less obvious foods, including confectionery and prepared foods.

If you are suffering from any type of depression we suggest that you avoid all wheat sources for at least a month. It is advisable to work with an experienced nutritional consultant to ascertain the level of wheat in your current diet and to identify practical – and palatable – alternatives.

NUTRITIONAL GUIDELINES FOR MANAGING DEPRESSION

1. Eat little and often to improve blood-sugar management.
2. Do not follow 'high-anything' diets (for example high-protein or high fat/high fibre diets); instead, eat a little from each food group at every meal and snack to ensure the maximum intake of all necessary nutrients.
3. Each a wide variety of foods.
4. Avoid stimulants such as caffeine, as it can lower absorption rates of the vital B vitamins.
5. Avoid alcohol, as it is a simple sugar, which can reduce mineral absorption, especially magnesium. It can also reduce absorption of nutrients in the colon.
6. Avoid wheat and wheat flour, as this over-used food may interfere with nutrient absorption in the small and large intestines.

A food allergy involves a swift response from the immune system, but food intolerances are more subtle and their effects are usually cumulative.

fatigue

Thyroid function

As we have seen (p.42), the gland that regulates our metabolic rate and energy production is the thyroid gland, which is situated at the base of the neck, near the Adam's apple. The pituitary gland in the brain releases a 'thyroid-stimulating hormone' to precipitate the production of thyroxine from the thyroid, which in turn regulates cellular metabolism. Poor thyroid function leads to lack of energy and low libido, and it may be worth getting the function of this gland checked if you have experienced recent weight gain plus loss of sexual interest and/or performance. Interestingly, a sudden change of menstruation in women can be attributable to a drop in thyroid function, rather than being an indication of the onset of menopause, so it is worth checking first before opting for HRT (hormone replacement therapy). Furthermore, poor thyroid function is associated with a drop in blood pressure, reducing the flow of blood to the sex organs in both men and women, and thereby resulting in fewer erections and lessening the ability to reach an orgasm.

THYROID STIMULATORS AND INHIBITORS

Foods that are rich in iodine, which is required by the thyroid for the production of thyroxine, are: kelp and other seaweeds, blue-green algae, shellfish and seafood, Swiss chard, kale, turnips and their greens, squash, watermelon, cucumber, spinach and okra.

Foods that inhibit thyroid function are mainly found in the brassica family of vegetables, namely broccoli, cauliflower, cabbage and Brussels sprouts. As these vegetables all contain important nutrients for other functions, we recommend that you reduce their intake, rather than eliminating them altogether.

Heart and cardiovascular problems

Heart disease is still the main cause of premature death in the Western world, and there are many kinds of heart problem from low blood pressure to angina.

A healthy heart and cardiovascular system is a prerequisite for stamina and a strong libido. Low blood pressure leads to mild or moderate fatigue, and may result in an inability to maintain an erection or become adequately aroused in the first place. Conversely, high blood pressure can present a problem during sex because normal blood pressure levels elevate naturally to ensure increased blood-flow to the sexual organs. In cases of severe hypertension, sexual activity can lead to palpitations, angina or chest pains.

Atherosclerosis is a condition in which the blood flow through the arteries becomes restricted due to a build-up of arterial plaque. This build-up is caused by particles of excess circulating cholesterol and calcium deposits binding together and attaching themselves to the artery walls. Atherosclerosis is associated with high blood pressure and may, in severe cases, lead to a restricted blood flow to the extremities. It is likely to inhibit sufficient blood flow to the sex organs in both men and women, reducing sensitivity and influencing arousal.

In numerous trials the antioxidant vitamins C and E have been found to protect arterial health. Eating plenty of berries, citrus fruits and watermelon, in addition to avocados, fresh nuts, seeds and wheatgerm, will help to maintain levels of these vital vitamins and encourage a healthy heart.

erectile dysfunction

Erectile dysfunction is thought to affect 30 million men in the West at one time or another. Although widespread, the problem – like most sexual problems – is rarely discussed.

With the advent of Viagra, however, the issue has come into the open, and the drug has proved remarkably popular, although it is generally preferable to discover the underlying cause of the problem, working to rebalance the body so that it does not recur. There are several natural alternatives to Viagra (see p.57), which some people may prefer to choose.

There are a number of possible causes of erectile dysfunction, including potential vascular disorders, neurological disorders, hormonal imbalances (testosterone deficiency, see p.54), diabetes, alcohol and drugs (see p.46).

The mechanism

To understand the interaction between nutrition and erectile function we must examine the mechanism of achieving and maintaining an erection. On stimulation from the brain, blood flow to the penis increases, forcing its sponge-like tissue to expand. This compresses minuscule veins, which act like taps, stopping the blood from flowing out of the penis, so that the tissue becomes engorged. Once the stimuli diminish, the veins slowly open, allowing blood to leave the tissue, which results in a return to flaccidity.

Obviously this mechanism depends heavily on blood flow, and increasing blood flow to the penis will therefore improve the erection. But blood flow is often compromised, especially with age, by atherosclerosis (see page 52). This can affect any part of the intricate series of arteries and capillaries that comprise the cardiovascular system. The condition is initiated by destructive molecules known as 'free radicals', which cause minute damage to the lining of the arteries. The body attempts to repair the damage by coating the affected area in a sticky plaque-type substance, but the internal circumference of the vessel then reduces, resulting in reduced blood flow to the affected area – in the case of erectile function, the genital region.

Nutritional support

The body protects itself from the potential damage caused by free radicals by creating substances known as antioxidants, but in order to produce enough antioxidants to quash the free radicals, there must be an adequate intake of various nutrients in the diet – namely the minerals zinc, selenium and magnesium and vitamins A, C and E.

Free-radical production is increased by a number of other factors, such as ultraviolet light, exercise (due to increased metabolic rate), smoking and fried foods. As free-radical production increases, so does the need for antioxidants. Damage is caused when the free radicals are not matched by antioxidant compounds. For this reason ensuring an optimum intake of nutrients that support this process is essential. Including fresh produce in the diet every day takes on added importance if you are unable to achieve or maintain an erection.

ANTIOXIDANT FOODS

The following foods are noted for their antioxidant properties:

FRUIT
apples, avocados, kiwi fruit, tomatoes, apricots, bananas, pears, blueberries, figs, blackcurrants, strawberries, lemons

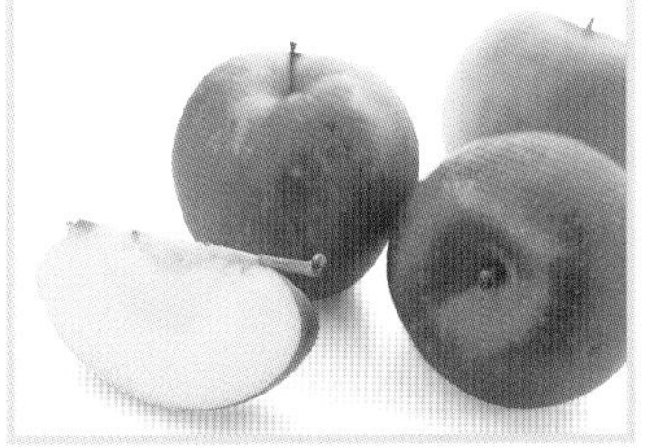

VEGETABLES
potatoes, chickpeas, kidney beans, asparagus, squashes, Brussels sprouts, carrots, onions and garlic, watercress , sweet potatoes, sea vegetables, beetroot (beet)

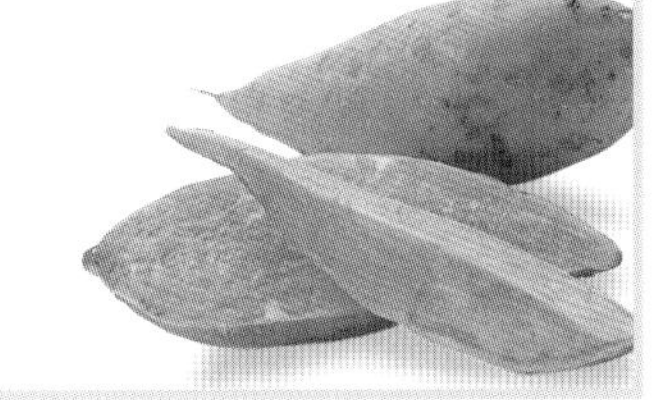

OTHERS
hazelnuts, sunflower, sesame and pumpkin seeds, parsley, spirulina, peanuts (raw), seafood (including tuna and salmon), chicken, grains (millet, oats, quinoa, rye, barley)

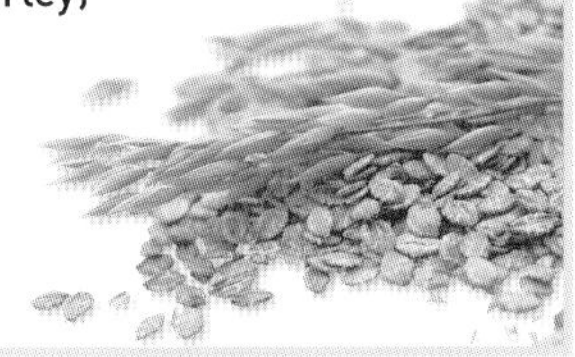

Recently other compounds have been identified as having powerful antioxidant properties. These include flavanols, proanthocyanins, polyphenols, carotenoids (such as lycopene, a constituent of tomatoes) and catechins. With the exception of catechins, which are found in tea, the rest are found in fruit and vegetables.

Blood-flow boosters

As we have seen, increasing blood flow to the penis is paramount in cases of erectile dysfunction. Many nutrients and herbs have been found to enhance blood flow, including gingko biloba, taken as a supplement; amounts of 60–80mg a day are thought to be optimal; co-enzyme Q-10 (see p. 21) has antioxidant properties, and is also known to enhance energy production; and vitamin E (see p. 23) thins the blood and can increase blood flow. It should not be taken if other blood-thinning agents (such as Warfarin) are being taken at the same time.

loss of libido in men

As we have seen, there are a number of factors that affect our libido and sexual appetite, including stress, depression, fatigue and heart and cardiovascular problems, but probably the most subtle element is hormonal imbalance (see p. 42) – in both men and women.

The sex hormones are intricately linked with the hormones released from the other endocrine glands throughout the body – all of which are connected by a feed-back loop mechanism. Adrenaline from the adrenal glands enables us to handle the myriad stresses of everyday life (see p. 44), while thyroxine in the thyroid gland regulates our metabolic rate and energy production (see p. 51). If either of these essential regulatory glands becomes overstressed, it will have a direct impact on the other glands, such as the ovaries and testes. Thus fatigue, anxiety and emotional pressures can become everyday stressors that underlie our loss of libido. Hence the all-too-frequent comments 'I'm too tired', or 'not tonight, darling'

Testosterone levels

Testosterone is present in both males and females and plays an important role in maintaining libido. In healthy men approximately 7mg of testosterone is produced daily by the Leydig cells in the testicles. However, stress has a direct effect on men, as the precursor hormones to both cortisol (the hormone that helps regulate the effects of stress) and testosterone originate from the same pathway. Imagine driving up to a T-junction and having to choose between turning left towards Managing Stress and turning right towards Producing Testosterone – the car will always go left first, if there is stress to be managed!

Testosterone plays an important role in maintaining libido.

Testosterone is fundamental to the production of sperm, fertility, erectile function and for regulating desire and libido. It also plays a part in preventing the onset of male osteoporosis. It is the reduction of testosterone that leads to the developing 'middle tyre' that is familiar to many middle-aged men – although this can happen earlier in men who

NUTRITIONAL REMEDIES

From a nutritional perspective, testosterone production is zinc- and vitamin B6-dependent. Nutritional deficiencies tend to increase with age, but zinc and vitamin B6 are both abundant in many of the foods we eat on a regular basis, so it is advisable to increase their intake.

ZINC-RICH FOODS
shellfish (especially oysters), sesame and pumpkin seeds, pine nuts, brown rice, cheese, seafood, eggs, lentils, chicken and turkey, spirulina, wholegrains

VITAMIN B6 FOODS
bananas, potatoes, chickpeas, chicken, tuna, avocados

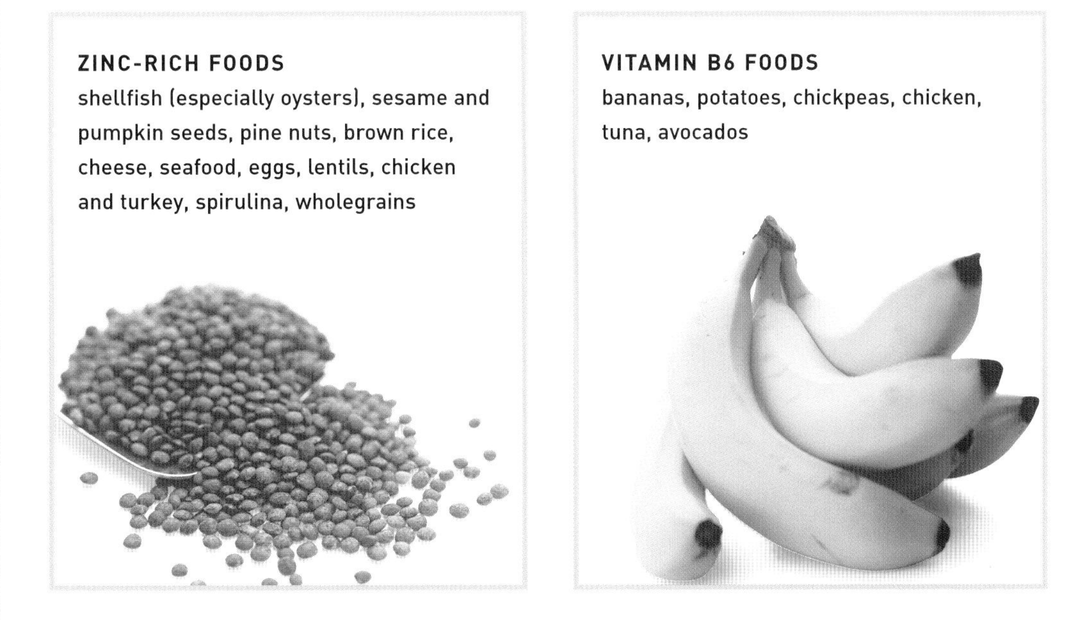

For both women and men, testosterone supplementation can be beneficial, either in the form of a patch or as a capsule (or occasionally given by injection). In all cases it is essential that base hormone levels are tested by a qualified doctor or endocrinologist, prior to undertaking any supplementation.

have engaged in stressful jobs and lifestyles, as increased adrenaline will reduce the production of testosterone.

Menopause – not just a female issue

It has long been acknowledged that the female menopause can have a profound impact on the mental and physical state of a woman in her forties and fifties. Less well known, however, is the status of a man during the same period of life, although it is now medically acknowledged that lowering levels of testosterone can affect men in much the same way. Much research has been carried out over the last few years to determine whether or not men, as well as women, experience a menopause. It has been noted that men appear to go through emotional as well as physical changes during their late forties to mid-fifties, such as experiencing a lack of goals and focus, an apparent loss of interest in family and close friends and lowered self-esteem, or even depression, in a similar pattern to that experienced by women. The male menopause is known as the viripause.

prostate health

Prostate health has recently become associated with erectile dysfunction, with prostate inflammation becoming so prevalent that many doctors see it as an almost unavoidable part of the ageing process for men. If you apply the appropriate nutritional guidelines then proper health can often be maintained.

The nut-sized prostate gland opens into the urethra (the channel leading from the bladder) and secretes a fluid that forms part of the semen. An enlarged prostate, or Benign Prostatic Hypertrophy (BPH), is common among men aged 20–60, and incidence increases with age (one-third of men over the age of 60 suffer from BPH), although it is still relatively rare in men under 45. When the prostate becomes enlarged, the neck of the bladder is obstructed, causing difficulties with urination. In some cases BPH can affect the ability to achieve an erection – one study showed that 44 per cent of men with BPH had difficulty in maintaining intercourse.

Conventional medicine often treats BPH surgically, or with drugs that reduce the gland's enlargement. One such drug was found to increase hair growth in balding men and has now been marketed as a remedy for baldness, not BPH. During the early stages of taking such drugs there is often a marked decrease in sexual desire, but this usually passes within eight weeks.

The prostate gland and nutrition

Studies have found that a diet high in saturated fats (found in red meat and dairy products, including milk) contributes to the incidence of BPH. Reducing your intake of these foods can improve the odds in your favour, but this does not mean following a low-fat diet. Most foods labelled 'low-fat' often contain increased levels of sugar to enhance their flavour, and while sugar in itself is not potentially damaging, it can lead to blood-sugar imbalances (see p. 40) and, more importantly, to increased production of insulin, which can have a mild pro-inflammatory effect. In

DIABETES AND ERECTILE DYSFUNCTION

There is a strong link between diabetes and erectile function. It has been estimated that impotence affects approximately 50 per cent of men with diabetes, and erectile dysfunction is now thought to be one of the early warning signs of the presence of diabetes.

Late-onset diabetes is the fastest-growing disease in the West, and this is attributable in no small part to our diets. We eat excessive amounts of simple carbohydrates (such as refined sugar and processed foods) and this, combined with a stressful lifestyle and other influences, means that more people than ever before are at risk of developing diabetes. If you already have the condition, then you are no doubt working with your doctor and are possibly taking insulin injections (subcutaneously). For those of us who do not, there are simple dietary measures that we can take to reduce our risk of developing late-onset diabetes. These include avoiding refined sugar – or reducing it as far as possible – and cutting down on stimulants such as caffeine and alcohol. Increasing our fibre intake (in the form of grains and dense vegetables) can also help, as can including a little protein at each meal and snack.

the case of the prostate gland, this can affect erection and urination (which may also interrupt sleep) and generally cause mild discomfort. Furthermore, the intake of certain fats is critical to our health. These 'essential fatty acids', or EFAs, must be derived from the diet, are found in oily fish, fresh nuts and their oils, linseeds and olive oil. EFAs are known to have an anti-inflammatory effect and have proved beneficial in cases of BPH.

The role of dietary oestrogens (isoflavonoids, flavonoids and lignins) has also been acknowledged in decreasing the incidence of BPH. It has been noted that BPH is less prevalent in Japan, and this is thought to be associated with the relatively high intake there of soya. Soya can be eaten in the form of tofu (a versatile and low-fat vegetarian protein source), soya milk, soya cheese and miso (fermented soya-bean paste).

Zinc (see p. 18) is also recommended to combat prostate problems, as men with BPH have been found to be deficient in this vital mineral. Include plenty of zinc-rich foods in your diet, and although getting nutrients from food is always preferable to supplementation, there is a strong argument for supplementing zinc for men with BPH. Doses of up to 50mg a day are thought to be safe, but ensure that you do not exceed 80mg of zinc from all sources (and other supplements you may be taking can contain zinc, so check the labels to ensure that you do not exceed safety levels).

the natural Viagra

Viagra has become one of the most sought-after medications during the last few years, as men of all ages have sought to increase their libido, or their stamina and staying power, and combat erectile dysfunction (see p. 52). Viagra works by increasing circulation to the penis, enabling an erection to be maintained. Potential problems lie in overuse, or use by those who have high blood pressure.

From a nutritional perspective, the amino acid L-arginine is regarded as the natural equivalent of Viagra. It is found in many protein foods of animal origin, particularly chicken, eggs, beef and dairy products, but may have to be taken as a supplement to produce the desired effect. It works by increasing the body's levels of a chemical called nitric oxide, which acts as a nerve transmitter, increasing blood flow to the penis. Contrary to the risk factors associated with high blood pressure and Viagra, L-arginine actually helps to regulate blood pressure and is therefore a potentially safer alternative. L-arginine can provoke herpes in the susceptible, so consult a qualified nutritional practitioner to assess if supplementation is appropriate and, if so, the correct levels.

There are periods in all our lives when our libido appears to have diminished, sometimes without tangible cause. If, however, you refer back to the Sex Questionnaire (see pp. 12–15), you will see from the sections on hormone disruption and stress that there are a number of experiences and lifestyle factors that have a direct effect on sexual appetite. Over the next few pages we shall examine the various reasons for loss of libido in women, and then look at how to boost your libido.

NATURAL ALTERNATIVES TO VIAGRA

SIBERIAN GINSENG

This herb (**Eleutherococcus senticosus**) is known to increase honey production in bees, sperm count in bulls and milk secretion in cows. It has been widely researched as an energy booster and as a means to increase stamina. It is also used to combat BPH.

YERBE MATE

This herbal tea, made from the bark of a tree (**Ilex paraguariensis**) native to Paraguay, is rich in minerals and vitamins (especially vitamin C). Its chief benefit is to support the adrenal glands during periods of stress – prolonged or chronic stress being known to interfere with the production of testosterone. Although Yerbe Mate is 97.7% caffeine free, it does contain small amounts of caffeine and therefore acts as a vasodilator, helping efficient blood flow. It also stimulates the adrenal glands which can boost short-term energy.

YOHIMBE

This substance stands out as being perhaps the most effective natural remedy for erectile dysfunction. Yohimbe is the bark from a tree (**Corynanthe yohimbe**) that grows in Zaïre and Cameroon. The bark contains substances that increase overall blood flow to the genital area. This has the effect of improving the strength both of the erection and of the subsequent ejaculation. Furthermore, yohimbe is reputed to stimulate the production of adrenaline and noradrenaline, which can enhance overall sensitivity.

Its efficacy has been proven in clinical trials, although some recent studies refute its potential benefits. However, it is very popular and users report excellent results, although with long-term use yohimbe has been reported to increase hypertension, so it should be treated with caution if you have high blood pressure. It can also contribute to strokes in susceptible individuals and other side-effects include headaches, anxiety and flushing. In the UK Yohimbe is restricted to sale by a registered pharmacy under supervision of a pharmacist. It is available in some European counties and in the United States, usually in a capsule or in the form of a tea, and should be used with caution.

Its relative effectiveness was underlined by widespread use of the drug Yohimbe Hydrochloride, which was prescribed in the US for erectile dysfunction before Viagra was available.

SARSAPARILLA

Originating from a climbing vine (**Smilax regelii**), sarsaparilla has hormone-like compounds that form the basis of several synthetic hormones, particularly testosterone, which is often lacking in men with erectile difficulties.

SAW PALMETTO

A palm tree (**Serenoa repens**) native to the West Indies, saw palmetto is widely used to combat inflammation and enlargement of the prostate. It is believed to contain substances that regulate hormonal stimulation of the prostate gland, which in turn can reduce overstimulation. Saw palmetto is widely available and there are few (if any) reported side-effects; it has been used with notable success in cases of BPH.

loss of libido in women

Dance of the hormones

In both men and women an intricate dance of hormones requires balancing in order to ensure regular and satisfactory sexual activity. Any disruption of these hormones may affect your sex drive, and it is important to understand which hormones direct your libido. Like men, women also produce testosterone (see p. 54), not just from their ovaries, but from their adrenal glands, brain, skin and fat stores as well. In fact these organs produce far more testosterone than the ovaries, and it is interesting to note that women who have spent their lives trying to stay thin often suffer far more during the menopause, as they have fewer fat stores of testosterone. Testosterone levels can be boosted by eating zinc-rich and vitamin B6 foods (see p. 55).

Imbalances of oestrogens and progesterone may also contribute to loss of libido, as the normal length of the menstrual cycle may be disturbed or lengthened. Women who suffer from bad PMS symptoms are far more likely to experience lack of sex drive than their unsuffering peers, as their physical and mental changes lead to mood swings and loss of self-esteem. The cycles of oestrogen and progesterone production and release are well understood under normal circumstances, but if either of these two essential hormones is not released at the correct time, various side-effects inevitably occur, affecting both your emotional and your physical status.

Oestrogen dominance is a common problem in the Western world today, affecting fertility, leading to an increased risk of ovarian and endometrial cancers, and being responsible for a large percentage of the breast cancers that are hormonally derived. Additionally, endometriosis and fibroids are the result of oestrogen dominance. The causes of such dominance are both environmental and dietary – many of our foods and the wrappings that we use to containerize our pre-packed foods incorporate oestrogen-like properties, which affect our circulating levels of this hormone. This interferes with the delicate balance and function of progesterone, encouraging weight gain, increased fat storage and exacerbated PMS symptoms, for which the traditional medical answer is usually...even more oestrogens! This is not a subject to be taken lightly, and the resulting loss of libido should be sufficient indication that other, more serious outcomes may follow, if it is not attended to.

Slave to your body

A woman's self-perception has a direct effect on her libido, and continuous representations of the 'perfect', slim-line figure have done untold harm to an inestimable number of women, for whom the term 'large' never previously acted as a deterrent to their sexuality. Endless diets inevitably lead to lowered metabolism, simply compounding the problems of weight management in the long term. A lowered metabolic rate equates with lack of energy, and hence with diminished libido.

Prescription and recreational drugs

Many prescription drugs have a libido-reducing effect. Most anti-depressants, for example, have a sedative effect, as may drugs prescribed for high blood pressure, raised cholesterol and other triglyceride imbalances. For a detailed description of how recreational drugs interfere with sexual behaviour, see p. 46.

Smoking and alcohol consumption should not be underestimated when evaluating libido-lowering agents. Smoking reduces oestrogen production in women and can lower sex drive – just as any amount of alcohol above one or two units per day causes female testosterone levels to rise sharply within a couple of hours of consumption and oestrogen levels to drop dramatically. The overall result is a lessening of vaginal secretions and lowered libido – a rather different picture from the 'release from inhibitions' that alcohol is supposed to bring.

SEX-BOOSTING NUTRIENTS AND HERBS

There are a number of herbs and other nutrients that have traditionally been used to support the female body, and research is now showing that the benefits they can bring constitute more than simply an old wives' tale.

EVENING PRIMROSE (OENOTHERA BIENNIS) OIL

Much is known about the role of evening primrose oil in the prevention and treatment of PMS, but it is important to understand that the same applies to sex drive. This valuable flower, from which the oil is extracted, is a rich source of GLA (gamma linolenic acid), one of the essential fatty acids, which is required for the production of sexual hormones. Research has shown that lowered sex drive resulting from fatigue is often improved by supplementation with evening primrose oil and other essential fatty acids, which help to boost cellular uptake of energy-enhancing nutrients. Rich sources of essential fatty acids include starflower and evening primrose oils, sesame, sunflower and pumpkin oils, walnut, linseed and flax oils. Adding some of these foods and oils to your daily diet is always beneficial.

BEE POLLEN AND ROYAL JELLY

Both of these are rich sources of amino acids, essential fatty acids, carbohydrates, minerals, vitamins and trace elements. Indeed, if a queen bee can live her entire life and lay thousands of eggs on a diet of royal jelly alone, perhaps more attention should be paid to her source of nutrition. Traditionally, both bee pollen and royal jelly (a substance secreted by worker bees and fed to all larvae, particularly those destined to become queens) are considered tonics for the whole body, when energy or strength has been lowered by stress or illness. Both are known to boost sex drive, and bee pollen is said to reduce hot flushes during the menopause. Rather than taking either substance on an ongoing basis, it is more effective to take them for one or two months at a time, with regular breaks in between. In some cases bee pollen or royal jelly can provoke an allergic reaction, in which case the course should be immediately halted.

BLUE-GREEN ALGAE

There is no known food source on the planet that contains a wider range of essential nutrients than blue-green algae – a power-house of nutrition that may be added to your daily diet to increase your energy levels and sex drive. Add it to milkshakes and smoothies, or to your favourite juice, for that health-giving 'green drink' boost.

Approaching the menopause

It is a well-known fact that the period of change in a woman's life, when her oestrogen and progesterone levels fall and regular menstruation ceases, is often a cause of lowered libido. As oestrogen levels drop, women often experience loss of self-esteem, a lack of direction in their lives and physical changes, including weight gain in the waist and hip areas, thickening of hair texture (both on the head and body) and thinning of the skin.

One of the most common problems relating to lower levels of oestrogen during the menopausal years is vaginal dryness, which causes itching, irritation and burning, sometimes even when there is

CHICKEN-EGG EXTRACTS

Owing to much inappropriate (and inaccurate) research that has indicated over the years that eating eggs can increase cholesterol levels, our consumption of this vital source of amino acids has dramatically declined. Eating battery-reared, unfertilized eggs may be part of the problem associated with lowered sex drive, but chicken-egg extracts (CEE) – taken from fertilized eggs – appeared to increase sex drive and sexual satisfaction in both men and women in a number of trials carried our recently, mainly in the United States. CEE are available in England under the tradename Libido, and are packaged in sachets of dissolving powders.

DONG QUAI OR DANG GUI (ANGELICA SINENSIS)

Containing oestrogen-like compounds, this adaptogen works by filling some of the oestrogen sites, to reduce the problems associated with oestrogen dominance in PMS. It also helps to relieve breast tenderness and menstrual cramps, as well as more serious problems such as endometriosis and fibroid formation, and provides additional oestrogen activity at the menopause. It can therefore boost women's sexual desire during either the premenstrual or menopausal phases, when loss of sex drive tends to be most severe. **Caution:** angelica can cause photo-sensitivity in some individuals and should therefore not be taken by women who have fair or freckly skin, or by those who burn easily in the sun. Best avoided if taking any blood-thinning agents, such as Warfarin.

CATUABA (JUNIPERUS BRASILIENSIS)

Noted for its sexual and erotic properties, this herb originated among the Tupi native peoples in Brazil, who used it as an aphrodisiac. It works as a stress-hormone adaptogen (that is, it balances the stress-managing mechanisms and hormones released from the adrenal glands) and has been found to be beneficial to women as well as men. Follow the manufacturers' instructions for correct dosages.

CHASTE BERRY (VITEX AGNUS-CASTUS)

Derived from a tree native to the Mediterranean and south-west Asia, this berry yields a substance that helps regulates hormones in women who are suffering from PMS or high prolactin levels (see below). It is not known to act directly on the relevant hormones, but rather affects dopamine levels in the brain, which can in turn alter sex drive. This herb is only suitable for women, as it has an androgen-lowering effect in men.

PROTECTIVE PHYTO-OESTROGENS

Phyto-oestrogens are oestrogen-like compounds found in specific foods that fill oestrogen receptor sites in certain tissues of the body and serve to increase the total number of circulating oestrogens in the body. The following foods may help to reduce the risk of osteoporosis (brittle bones), as well as increase libido and regulate weight gain during the menopause.

linseeds, soya products, fennel, oats, sunflower seeds, pumpkin seeds, celery, barley, sesame seeds, poppy seeds, red onions, brown rice, red grapes, citrus fruit, broccoli, rye, chickpeas, cranberries, sweet peppers, polenta, kidney beans, cherries, tomatoes, buckwheat, mung beans, watermelon, garlic, raspberries

no sexual activity. For some women, this is a cause of great concern. Lubricating creams and lotions can offer some relief, but it is more important to try to increase phyto-oestrogens in your diet.

Prolactin in pregnancy

The hormonal changes that occur during and after pregnancy can also have detrimental effects on libido. In fact, some women lose their libido completely after giving birth. This is probably due to another hormone, prolactin, which is produced by the hypothalamus in the brain. Prolactin stimulates breast milk, and is restricted by a neurotransmitter in the brain, known as dopamine. Dopamine also drives, indirectly, the levels of testosterone production, so if a woman is breastfeeding, her prolactin levels will be high and her testosterone levels low. In some cases, however, the prolactin does not switch itself off. This can be one of the side-effects of anti-depressants such as Prozac, which works on another neurotransmitter (serotonin) sitting on the other end of the seesaw from dopamine. If serotonin levels are high, then dopamine levels will be lower, causing less production of testosterone and hence reduced libido. One herb that can be used to balance dopamine levels (and hence reduce high levels of prolactin) is chaste berry (see p.61).

libido boosters

We have looked in depth at the various causes for loss of libido, including hormonal problems of several kinds. As we have shown, all of these negative aspects can be addressed through diet and lifestyle choices. In addition, there are specific vitamins and other nutrients (described below) that can boost libido in both men and women. For added information on essential minerals refer to Nutritional Deficiencies (pages 18–21).

BETWEEN THE SHEETS (OR LIBIDO-BOOSTERS)

NUTRIENT	FUNCTION	RICHEST SOURCES
VITAMIN A	Important for regulating sexual growth by stimulating specific genes in response to sex-hormone triggers. It is also vital for the production of oestrogen and testosterone. There are two forms of vitamin A: retinol (found in animal produce) and beta-carotene (the precursor to retinol, converted from vegetable sources).	Retinol: the livers of animals, all dairy produce, eggs and oily fish. Beta-carotene: dark green leafy vegetables and yellow-orange fruits.
VITAMIN B-COMPLEX	The B group of vitamins is important for the production of energy – without which there is no libido worth talking about. Vitamin B6 plays a regulatory role in sex-hormone function and Vitamin B3 induces an increase in the flexibility of the capillary walls of the circulatory system, causing them to dilate and allowing more blood to the area.	Wholegrains (especially brown rice) and cereals, pulses, nuts, yeast extracts, meat, fish, eggs, dairy produce, avocados, cream, mushrooms and broccoli.
VITAMIN C	Vitamin C is essential for increasing semen volume, and for ensuring that sperm do not clump together. It also has the capability to boost sex drive and strengthen the sex organs in both men and women.	Raspberries, blackberries, strawberries, citrus fruit, kiwi fruit, mangoes, papayas, figs, potatoes, green peppers, broccoli, beetroot (beet) and sprouted vegetables.
VITAMIN E	Vitamin E is involved in the manufacture of sex hormones, and a deficiency of this protective vitamin is associated with low sex drive and reduced fertility.	Oily fish such as salmon, tuna, sardines and herring, liver, eggs and dairy produce.
CHROMIUM	A lack of chromium will affect your blood-sugar management and energy levels; more specifically, a deficiency of chromium decreases sperm count and sex drive.	Wholegrains and cereals, meat, cheese, yeast and thyme.
BORON	Boron is a trace element, and yet it is vital for the production of sex hormones. Minute amounts of this mineral will increase both oestrogen and testosterone levels.	All fruit and vegetables.

part two: **sleep**

sleep

Foods to improve the quality of your sleep

why sleep is

It is fast becoming accepted that we live in a sleep-deprived age, where the importance of achievement in both our working and home lives necessitates being awake and alert for as many hours in the day as possible – but at what cost to our bodies? It is only during sleep that we are able to rebuild ourselves, using the amino acids derived from the proteins that we eat during the day. A specific stage of sleep, known as REM (Rapid Eye Movement, see below) sleep, enables our immune system to produce more immune cells, and without this vital stage of sleep, that system inevitably falters and lowers its protection.

The balance of wakefulness and sleep is regulated by the production of two corticosteroids from the adrenal glands, cortisol (see p.96) and adrenaline (see p.95). These two hormones are responsible for waking us up in the morning, as well as being the primary hormones that regulate stress. When someone is overstressed and these hormones are being produced regularly throughout the day, then they become exhausted and their ability to wake that person up in the morning is therefore reduced. Feeling tired in the morning is one of the primary signs of adrenal fatigue.

THE FUNCTION OF SLEEP

Sleep has various benefits for the body, but its main functions are:

1. **The release of human growth hormone, which is produced in the pituitary gland, stimulates the rebuilding of our organs and tissues while our bodies rest.**
2. **Lowering the body's metabolic rate to ensure that the catabolism (breaking down) of organ cells is reduced, and that energy is not released in the same quantity as during the day.**
3. **Lessening the need for oxygen, allowing the lungs to function more rhythmically, and with fewer demands on the body.**
4. **Building immunity by stimulating the production of immune cells from bone marrow.**
5. **Psychologically, absorbing the experiences of the day, to add to the brain's library of information and knowledge, and filing the facts appropriately. Dreams are merely an extension of the way in which we choose to store and file our perceived experiences. Inadequate sleep prevents us from doing this and may lead to distorted perception of both ourselves and others.**

good for you

SLEEP PATTERNS (PHASES OF SLEEP)

All sleep falls into two main phases: REM, or orthodox sleep, and non-REM, or paradox sleep. Rapid Eye Movement sleep only constitutes approximately 20 per cent of the time spent asleep. Non-REM sleep falls into four separate sub-categories:

STAGE 1 drowsiness (book on your nose phase) – it is during this stage that your body often jerks or jumps (known as hypnagogic startle)

STAGE 2 light sleep (a knock on the door would still wake you up)

STAGE 3 medium sleep (you are unlikely to hear movement outside your room)

STAGE 4 heavy sleep (you won't hear a thing!) – it is during this stage that your breathing patterns and heartbeat become most stable and slow down.

REM sleep occurs sporadically during the non-REM cycle, but the following physical changes are noticeable. The body's metabolic rate speeds up, as does breathing, and the eyeballs are seen to be moving rapidly under the eyelids. It is during this stage that we dream, and from this stage that we usually wake, or partially awaken before starting the whole cycle again. Interestingly, the nerve impulses emanating from the spine are virtually blocked during this stage, creating total relaxation in the muscles and limiting movement. This explains why some people wake from dreaming or having a nightmare saying that they felt they were immobilized.

The length of sleep cycles varies from child to adult. The average length of a sleep cycle in a baby is 50 minutes, which is extended to approximately 90 minutes by adolescence. This explains the necessity for a minimum of six hours, and preferably nine hours, of sleep per night in order to ensure several complete phases of sleep. Inadequate sleep has both short- and long-term ramifications, as we shall see later on (pp.98–9).

The questionnaire on pp.68–71 will enable you to establish how efficiently you are sleeping, and what areas of your diet and lifestyle may need attending to. The foods and herbs listed in the section on Sleepy foods (pp.78–85) have various roles to play. It may surprise you to find that some foods that you might previously have thought of as heavy or unsuitable for night-time actually contain specific nutrients that contribute to a restorative night's sleep.

sleep questionnaire

There are many factors that affect our quality of sleep, and all of us go through periods of lighter or interrupted sleep at different points in our lives. It is well known that we need less sleep as we get older, which is related to the slower pace of the rebuilding of our bodies as the years advance. However, resting or light napping is also beneficial, and should not be overlooked. Look through the following questionnaire and answer those questions that seem applicable to you, to gauge your own sleep efficiency. There is no scoring system – the questionnaire is designed to raise your awareness of possible contributory factors, so that you can relate the following sections to your own lifestyle.

HORMONE DISRUPTION

Hormones, the chemical messengers that control our body functions, also regulate the body's circadian rhythm (or 24-hour clock, see p.94), as well as stress (see p.95) and mood, so hormonal disruption can have major repercussions on our sleep patterns. Stress plays the greatest role in disrupting hormones, as every system in the body is affected.

FEMALE

1. Are you currently taking HRT (hormone replacement therapy)?
2. Are you taking any medication for sleeping, or anti-depressants?
3. Do you suffer from breast tenderness?
4. Is there a history of breast/ovarian/uterine cancer in your family?
5. Have you experienced amenorrhoea (cessation of regular menstruation) at any time in the last five years?
6. Do you have an excessive growth of body hair?

MALE

1. Are you experiencing hair loss or a receding hairline?
2. Has your weight distribution increased around your midline (abdomen)?
3. Do you have a noticeably lower sex drive than you used to?
4. Have you experienced any unexplained weight gain over the last few years?
5. Are you currently taking any medication for hypertension, any anti-depressants or tranquillizers?
6. Have you noticed a change in the production of your body hair or facial hair?
7. Have you taken steroid medication for asthma, eczema or other inflammatory conditions for more than two years?

BLOOD-SUGAR MANAGEMENT

Energy production throughout the day, as well as our ability to relax and have a good night's sleep, is dependent on the way we digest and absorb our food. Balancing blood-sugar levels and preventing fluctuations (see p.97) is one of the key elements in preventing insomnia and other sleep problems.

1 Do you suffer from bouts of fatigue throughout the day?
2 Do you have frequent sugar cravings?
3 Do you often have an unquenchable thirst?
4 Do you easily become irritable or angry?
5 Do you tolerate others poorly?
6 Do you feel fatigued towards the end of the day?
7 Do you wake up feeling the need for more sleep?
8 Do you sometimes feel dizzy and light-headed?
9 Are you prone to fainting?
10 Do you rely on coffee/ tea to keep you going throughout the day?
11 Is there a history of diabetes in your family?

TOXICITY

Once they have accumulated in our bodies, toxins affect the delicate balance of neurotransmitters that dictate when we sleep and when we wake. A degree of environmental pollution is inevitable, but there are certain toxins over which we do have some control, such as the stimulants of caffeine (found not only in coffee, tea, chocolate and carbonated drinks but in some medicines, see p. 100, alcohol and drugs).

1 Do you smoke more than five cigarettes daily?
2 Do you drink alcohol daily?
3 Do you take recreational drugs?
4 Are you on any prescription medication?
5 Do you have amalgam fillings in your teeth?
6 Do you live in a busy, built-up area?
7 Are you excessively exposed to car and transport fumes?
8 Do you work in the airline industry?
9 Do you spend long hours in front of the television or a VDU?
10 Do you work in an industry that requires you to come into contact with chemicals, either handled or inhaled?
11 Do you live close to either electricity pylons or mobile telephone masts?
12 Do you use a cellphone for extended periods?

DIETARY FACTORS

Good diet is obviously important for overall health and essential for maintaining the body (remember that rebuilding occurs during sleep). Many incorrect or unsuitable dietary choices can seriously affect our quality of sleep – for instance, the timing, quantity and quality of our food intake (see p.100), as well as drastic cycles of dieting and eating (see p.100).

1. Do you consume a large percentage of processed, ready-prepared meals?
2. Do you eat fried food regularly?
3. Do you suffer from constipation?
4. Do you take antacid medication for indigestion?
5. Do you consume more than two cups of tea/coffee per day?
6. Do you drink more than two units of alcohol daily?
7. Do you experience bloating on a regular basis?
8. Do you suffer from wind/flatulence?
9. Is your diet rich in dairy produce?
10. Do you often consume canned carbonated drinks?
11. Do you often snack on packet foods?
12. Do you have a high intake of chocolate and confectionery?

EMOTIONAL FACTORS

Our emotional state has a direct bearing on the quality of our sleep, and we often take our problems to bed with us, rather than trying to relax or save the problem-solving for tomorrow. Yet being tired compounds the problem and can increase feelings of depression, which may be linked to low serotonin levels, and be both the cause and effect of insomnia (see p.99).

1. Are you generally unhappy with your life at present?
2. Are you currently on your own, and lonely?
3. Do you seem to suffer from frequent bouts of anger and irritability?
4. Are you going through the menopause (male or female)?
5. Have you recently lost someone close to you?
6. Have you just separated/divorced from your partner?
7. Have you recently had a child?
8. Have you moved home or job?
9. Are you suffering from a lack of self-esteem?
10. Are you currently in an unsuitable and/or unsatisfactory relationship?

STRESS

Stress is inextricably linked to anxiety and tension (see p.99), and it affects our levels of continuity of sleep. It is also linked to blood-sugar levels, because when the body is stressed a hormone called cortisol is released, increasing blood-sugar levels and causing insomnia. Check the following questions to see which stresses may be affecting you.

1. Do you find it difficult to relax when you have time off?
2. Do you never manage to take time out each day from your busy schedule?
3. Do you carry out several tasks simultaneously?
4. Do you lose your temper easily?
5. Do you often forgo exercise due to fatigue or a hectic schedule?
6. Do you fly transatlantically or long-distance more than once a month?
7. Do you suffer from insomnia?
8. Do you often work late?
9. Do you wake feeling unrested and in need of more sleep?
10. Do you often wake in the middle of the night?

HEART HEALTH

Heart and cardiovascular problems have a profound effect on our quality of sleep and are associated with problems such as sleep apnoea (see p.104). Palpitations, high blood pressure and angina all affect our depth of sleep and sleep patterns. Unfortunately our lifestyles and eating habits often impede optimum heart health, but there is plenty that we can do to improve the situation.

1. Have you experienced angina or severe heart pain recently?
2. Do you find yourself short of breath after climbing a flight of stairs?
3. Are you less fit than you used to be?
4. Is your blood pressure higher than 120/75?
5. Do you take regular exercise that raises your heartbeat for more than 20 minutes?
6. Do you have cold hands and feet?
7. Do you have poor circulation?
8. Do you suffer from varicose or thread veins?
9. Do you experience palpitations?
10. Do you add salt to your food?

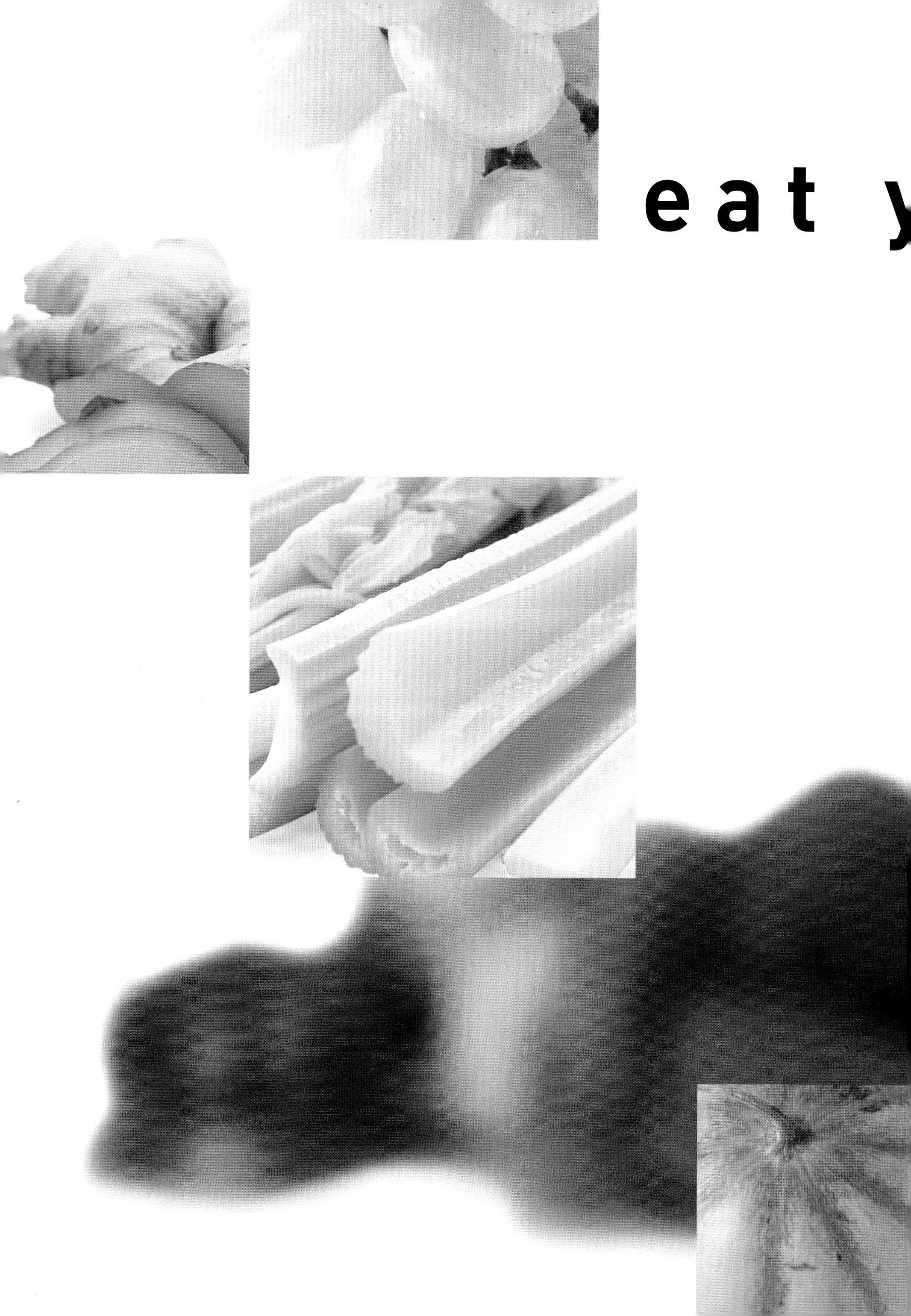
e a t y

our way to better sleep

foods to improve the quality of your sleep

There are numerous factors that affect the length and quality of our sleep. Eating habits are often overlooked but we feel that they contribute to sleep problems more than any other single factor.

The old adage 'breakfast like a king, lunch like a queen and dine like a pauper' holds true. Our circadian rhythms (see pages 94–95) function synergistically with this method of eating because our digestive capabilities are at their optimum levels in the early part of the day.

There is no doubt that our food choices, particularly in the latter part of the day, can affect the quality of our sleep. Many foods are known to have a sedative effect but there are also an abundance of foods that have a stimulatory effect.

In the following pages we look at the specific nutrients required for the promotion of regular, sound and restorative sleep. Any imbalance of these nutrients may induce minor sleep problems, so it is worth paying attention to the specific foods that will encouarge better sleep for you.

nutritional deficiencies

Some very specific nutrients are needed for the promotion of sound and restorative sleep. Look at each of the following groups of questions separately. If you answer 'yes' to three or more questions in any one group, it is possible that you are deficient in that mineral, vitamin or nutrient. The 'Richest Sources' box will tell you what foods you require.

IRON	FUNCTION	RICHEST SOURCES
• Do you tire easily? • Do you have pale skin? • Do you get out of breath easily? • Do you feel dizzy after mild exertion? • Are you slow to heal? • Do you suffer from heavy periods?	**Iron** is needed for the absorption of vitamin C, which must be consumed daily, since it cannot be stored by the body. It is also essential for the formation of the red pigment (haemoglobin) in blood, which carries oxygen throughout the body and ensures that the brain receives sufficient oxygen, both during sleep and in waking hours.	Liver, red meat, chicken, caviar, raisins, prunes, apricots, figs, egg yolks, wholegrains, watercress, spinach, broccoli, beetroot (beet), artichokes and pulses.

MAGNESIUM	FUNCTION	RICHEST SOURCES
• Do you get muscle cramps? • Do you have problems getting to sleep or staying asleep? • Are you easily startled? • Do you have problems relaxing? • Do you suffer from bad menstrual cramps? • Do you experience muscle weakness, tiredness or pain? • Do you become easily fatigued? • Do you suffer from anxiety/nervousness? • Do you often get cramp when exercising?	**Magnesium** is required for the absorption of calcium. It is known as the 'relaxation mineral', since it is the primary mineral required by the adrenal glands to help the body cope with stress (see p.44), as well as being a muscle-relaxant. Insomnia (see p.98) and other sleep problems (see p.102) often arise from an overstressed body and mind, so a high intake of magnesium-rich foods can help to counteract these problems.	Green leafy vegetables, lettuce, beetroot (beet), pumpkin, sweet potatoes, nuts, cheese, bananas, apricots, peaches, cereal grains, caviar, tuna and seafood.

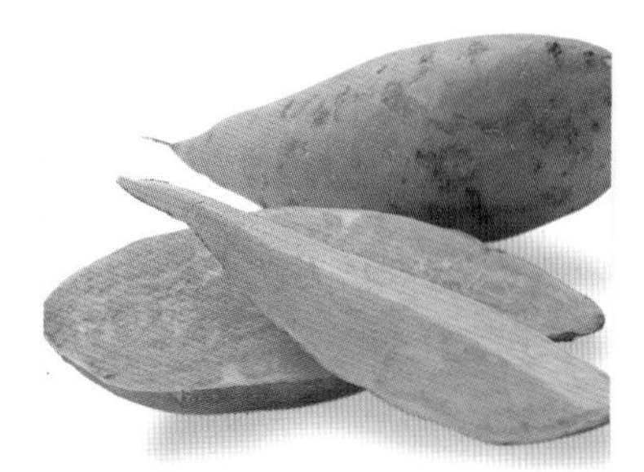

CALCIUM	FUNCTION	RICHEST SOURCES
• Do you suffer from insomnia or other sleep problems? • Are you nervous and jumpy? • Do you experience unexplained tingling sensations in your arms or legs? • Do you occasionally have muscle twitches? • Do you suffer from arthritic pain? • Do you have poor dental health? • Do you ever experience heart palpitations or a missed heartbeat?	**Calcium** is required in balance with magnesium, calcium regulates the heartbeat and blood pressure, and it is known that high blood pressure can interfere with the five different stages of sleep. Calcium also plays a part in nerve transmission, including potentiating (increasing the effectiveness of) the chemicals that transmit mood and relaxation, which are known as neurotransmitters.	Dairy products (including plain yoghurt), eggs, green leafy vegetables, beetroot (beet), pumpkin, watercress, kidney beans, prunes, apples, peaches, buckwheat, barley, sunflower seeds, nuts, turkey, tuna, shellfish and small fish that are eaten whole (e.g. sardines and whitebait). 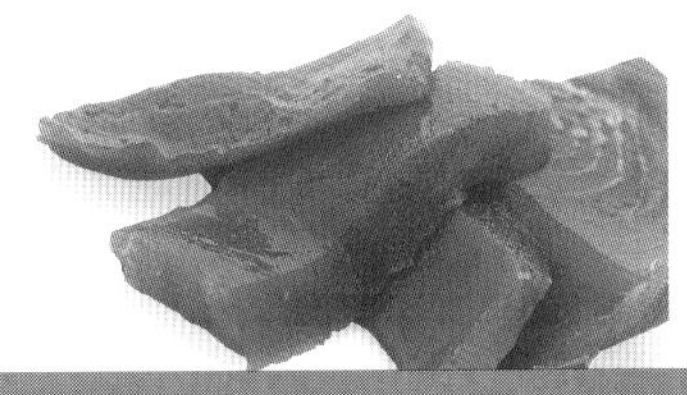

COPPER	FUNCTION	RICHEST SOURCES
• Do you have pale skin? • Do you tire easily? • Do you have poor skin texture or elasticity? • Do you have a high cholesterol level? • Do you suffer from arrhythmia (an abnormal heart rhythm)? • Do you have high blood pressure? • Do you suffer from energy fluctuations throughout the day?	**Copper** works in tandem with iron in the production of red blood cells to ensure that adequate oxygen is delivered to the brain during sleep as well as waking hours. It is also involved in blood-sugar management (see p.97), heightened cholesterol levels and high blood pressure. Deficiencies can occur from excessive zinc supplementation, as the two work synergistically and diametrically in the body.	Oysters and crabs, fish, nuts, lentils, oats, bananas, white beans and dark green vegetables. 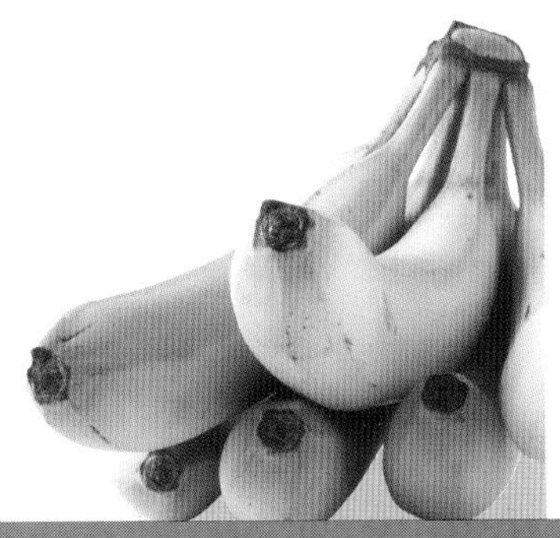

CHROMIUM	FUNCTION	RICHEST SOURCES
• Are you overweight for your height? • Do you have a need to urinate frequently? • Do you sometimes suffer from urinary infections? • Are you excessively thirsty? • Do you suffer from mood fluctuations? • Do you occasionally feel dizzy if you haven't eaten in several hours?	**Chromium** is primarily required for blood-sugar management (see p.97), as it potentiates the production and release of insulin. Insufficient chromium in the diet prevents effective blood-sugar control, which in turn interferes with the normal 90-minute sleep pattern, causing waking in the middle of the night or interrupted sleep.	fish, chicken, beef, dairy products, cheese, wholegrains and fruit. 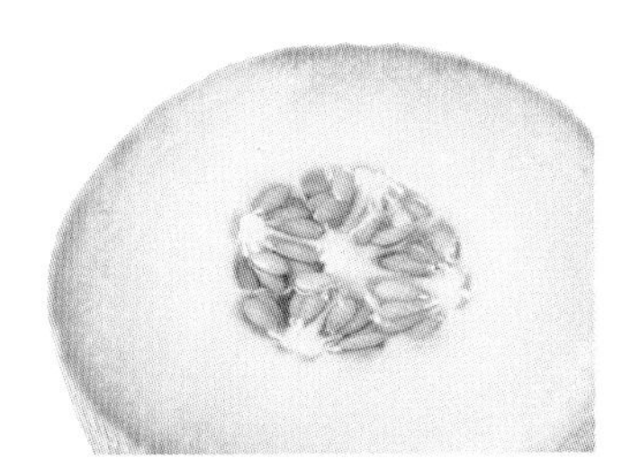

Essential fatty acids (EFAs)	FUNCTION	RICHEST SOURCES
• Do you suffer from dry skin? • Do you have stretch-marks? • Do you have small bumps or spots on the back of your arms? • Do you have cracked nails, dry hair or peeling lips? • Is the skin on your lower legs dry or creased? • Do you have a thickening of the skin on the heels and/or soles of your feet? • Are you prone to premenstrual tension? • Do you respond slowly to events? • Do you suffer from dyslexia?	**EFAs** are split into two main groups – omega-3 and omega-6 – and are known as 'essential' because they must be derived from the diet, since the body cannot manufacture them. They are responsible for nerve transmission from one nerve cell to another to regulate sleep patterns, and ensure balanced neurotransmitters during sleeping and waking.	Omega-3 EFAs: fish and seafood (including tuna, sardines and halibut), almonds, pine nuts, sesame, sunflower and pumpkin seeds and their oils; omega-6 EFAs: avocados, almonds, pine nuts, pumpkin, sunflower, sesame, linseed and hemp seeds and their oils.

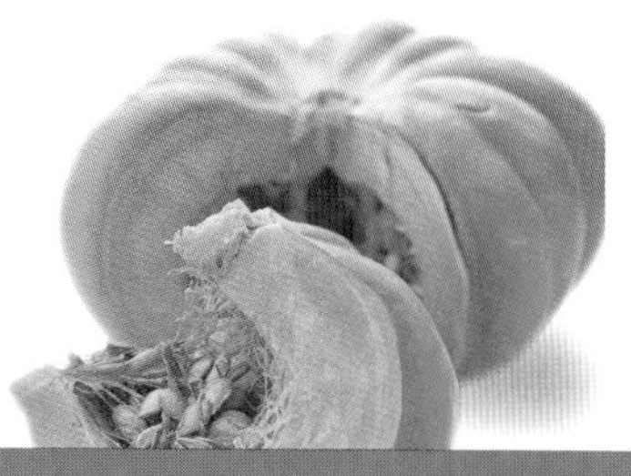

VITAMIN C	FUNCTION	RICHEST SOURCES
• Do you suffer from regular colds or other infections? • Do you have poor skin texture or elasticity? • Do you suffer regularly from bleeding gums? • Do you bruise easily? • Do you have nosebleeds? • Are you slow to heal? • Do you experience intermittent sleep disruption? • Do you have arterial or venous problems, such as varicose veins?	**Vitamin C** cannot be stored in the body, so it is imperative that we consume it through our diet on a daily basis, as it enables so many of our body systems to function optimally. Vitamin C is required for the conversion of tryptophan to serotonin (see p.95), the neurotransmitter that regulates our sleep, as well as being important for heart health.	Raspberries, blackberries, cherries, blueberries, citrus fruit, apples, kiwi fruit, peaches, mangoes, papayas, pineapple, figs, potatoes, sweet potatoes, green peppers, broccoli, beetroot (beet) and sprouted vegetables, such as mung beans and alfalfa sprouts.

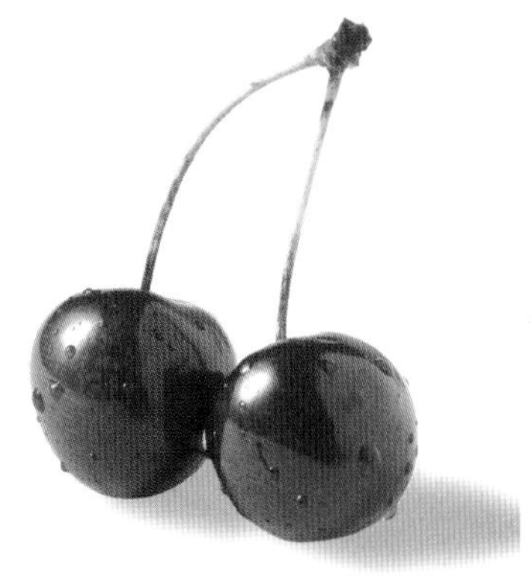

VITAMIN B-COMPLEX
including B1, B2, B3, B5, B6, B12, folic acid

- Is your memory or concentration as good as it used to be?
- Do you suffer from bouts of depression?
- Do you have cracked lips/split nails/bleeding or tender gums?
- Are you exhausted after exercise?
- Do you have digestive problems?
- Are you prone to anxiety and/or tension?
- Do you grind your teeth?
- Do you suffer from skin complaints (eczema, psoriasis, etc.)?

FUNCTION

B-complex vitamins are involved in all aspects of energy production at a cellular level, as well as in digestion and absorption. They are necessary for the regulation of mood and self-perception, motivation and relaxation.

Vitamin B3 is needed to ensure balanced blood-sugar management (see p.97) in order to prevent insomnia (see p.98) and interrupted sleep.

Vitamin B5 is required by the adrenal glands to regulate the body against the effects of long-term stress (see p.95). It also helps the body to cope with inadequate sleep in the short term.

Vitamin B6 is essential for mood enhancement and relaxation, being a co-factor of tryptophan conversion to serotonin (see p.95) – vital for promoting good sleep. It is also required to combat many of the symptoms of PMS. And choline is the precursor to acetyl-choline – the neurotransmitter required for the transmission of nerve impulses, which enhances mood and helps create the 'feel-good' factor.

RICHEST SOURCE

Wholegrains (especially brown rice) and cereals, pulses, tofu, nuts, sunflower seeds, yeast extracts, beef, fish, chicken, eggs, dairy produce, avocados, apricots, asparagus, potatoes, mushrooms, pak choi and broccoli.

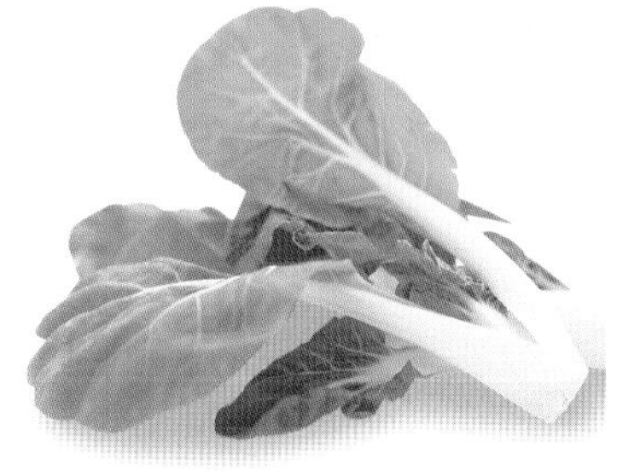

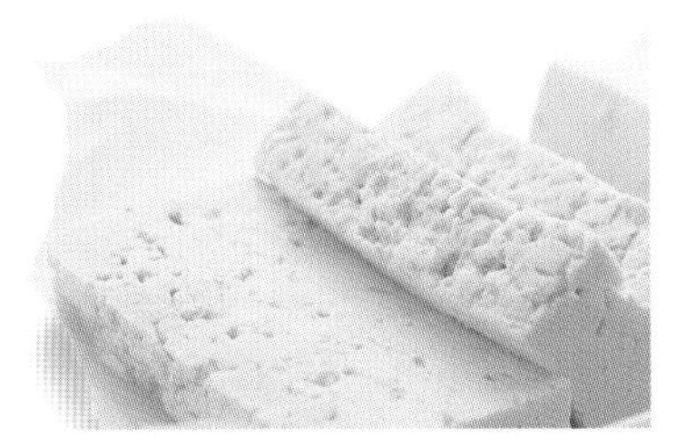

sleepy foods

There are numerous foods that either contain specific substances that enhance sleep, or that will combat commonly experienced problems that keep you awake. The following forty sleepy foods will help you to achieve a perfect night's sleep.

Seaweed — zzzz

More widely available in recent years, and a delicious accompaniment to many dishes (aside from Japanese cooking), seaweed (including kelp) is rich in tryptophan, the essential amino acid that is involved in melatonin production (see p.95).

beta-carotene, iodine, tryptophan, B vitamins

Sweet potatoes — zz

High in both magnesium and vitamin C, sweet potatoes have a good level of fibre to help regulate blood-sugar management (see p.97). This makes them an ideal base for thick, comforting soups and stews for evening meals.

magnesium, vitamin C

Beetroot (beet) — zzzz

High in both calcium and magnesium, this ruby-red vegetable provides a perfect balance for a good night's sleep. It is also a rich source of iron and vitamin C. Beetroot (beet) is also a good food for those suffering from chronic fatigue syndrome/ME. It may be eaten raw, juiced or cooked in a variety of ways.

calcium, iron, magnesium, vitamin C

Beef — zzzz

Beef is a rich source of both tryptophan and vitamin B3, which work together in the body to reduce anxiety, create calm and induce sleep. It is also a rich source of iron and chromium. The World Health Organization (WHO) recommends, however, that beef should not be eaten more than a few times each month.

chromium, iron, tryptophan, B vitamins

z Each z represents a sleepy nutrient.

Lettuce zzz

Although high in water content, lettuce is rich in magnesium to aid relaxation, and contains an opium-like compound called latucin, that encourages good sleep. It may be eaten raw in salads or lightly wilted with another vegetable, such as spinach, to increase the total nutrient value.

calcium, magnesium, vitamin C

Pumpkin zzzzz

Most vegetables contain some calcium and magnesium, but pumpkins have a particularly high balance of both of these minerals. They also contain abundant fibre, to help balance blood-sugar levels (see p.97). They may be used in casseroles and soups or roasted/baked as a vegetable side-dish. Pumpkin seeds are rich in omega-3 and omega-6 EFAs.

calcium, magnesium, omega-3 and omega-6 EFAs (in the seeds), vitamin C

Tuna zzzzzz

One of the most nutritious foods, tuna contains abundant calcium, magnesium and omega-3 EFAs to support the nervous system and allow the transmission of the essential neurotransmitters responsible for inducing good-quality sleep. It is a source of copper and chromium, both important for blood-sugar managements and is also a rich in B-complex vitamins, which are required for stress reduction. Tinned as well as fresh tuna provides these important nutrients.

calcium, chromium, copper, magnesium, omega-3 EFAs, B vitamins

Globe artichokes zzzzz

One of the highest vegetable sources of iron is found in artichokes, promoting a good supply of oxygen to the brain. It is believed that lack of oxygen is one of the main causes of sleep apnoea (where breathing stops temporarily during sleep, see p.104), so an increase of iron in the diet may be beneficial for this particular problem.

calcium, iron, magnesium, vitamins B3 and C

Broccoli — zzz

Considered one of the 'superfoods' for its potential role in cancer protection and its other antioxidant properties, broccoli is rich in B-complex vitamins, especially B3. It also contains iron and abundant vitamin C (see p.76), all of which ensure good oxygen flow to the brain.

iron, vitamins B and C

Avocados — zzzzz

Another 'superfood', avocado is rich in the B group of vitamins, particularly B6. It is also an excellent source of EFAs – rather than saturated fats, with which it is often associated. It may be eaten on its own, made into guacamole or added to a range of salads and cold soups.

copper, iron, omega-3 EFAs, vitamins B and E

Rye — zzz

This complex carbohydrate forms the basis of many breads and crackers, and makes a good source of the B-complex vitamins, in particular B3. It contains less gluten than wheat, so may be useful for those who show an intolerance to gluten.

calcium, iron, B vitamins

Turkey — zz

Turkey is one of the most abundant sources of tryptophan to encourage relaxation and sound sleep, so it is little wonder that most people find themselves more than usually tired after a Christmas or Thanksgiving dinner! Turkey is also high in calcium, and is regularly eaten with vegetables that possess plenty of magnesium, thereby providing the correct balance of these two minerals that are essential for preventing insomnia (see p.98).

calcium, tryptophan

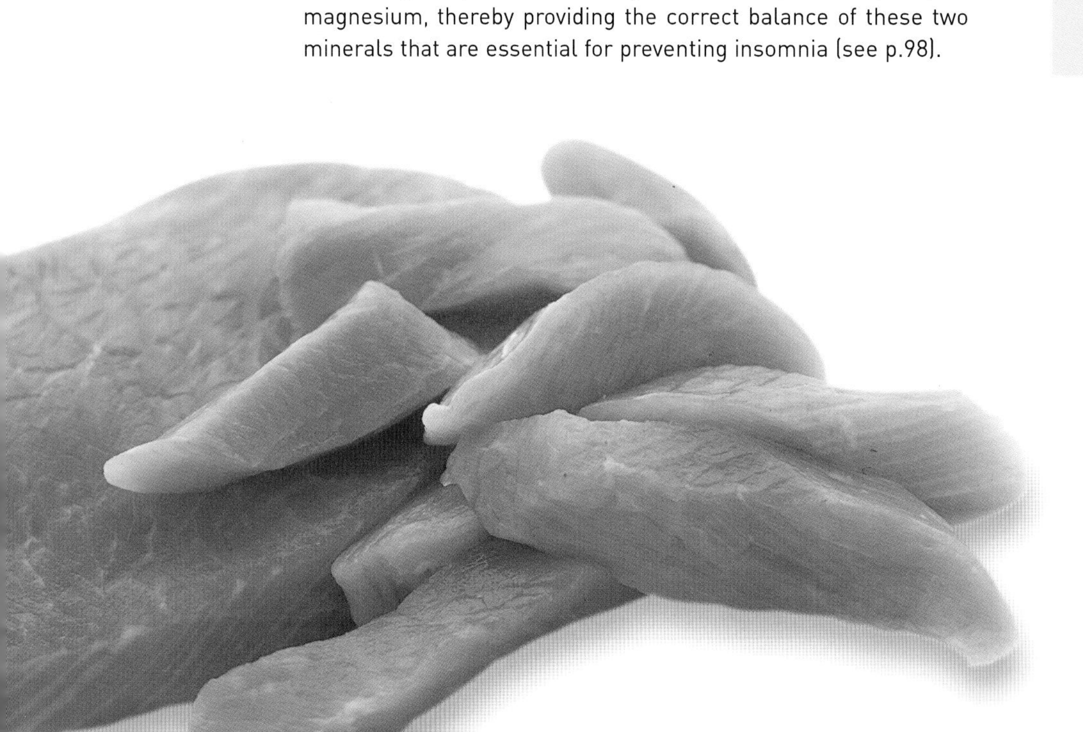

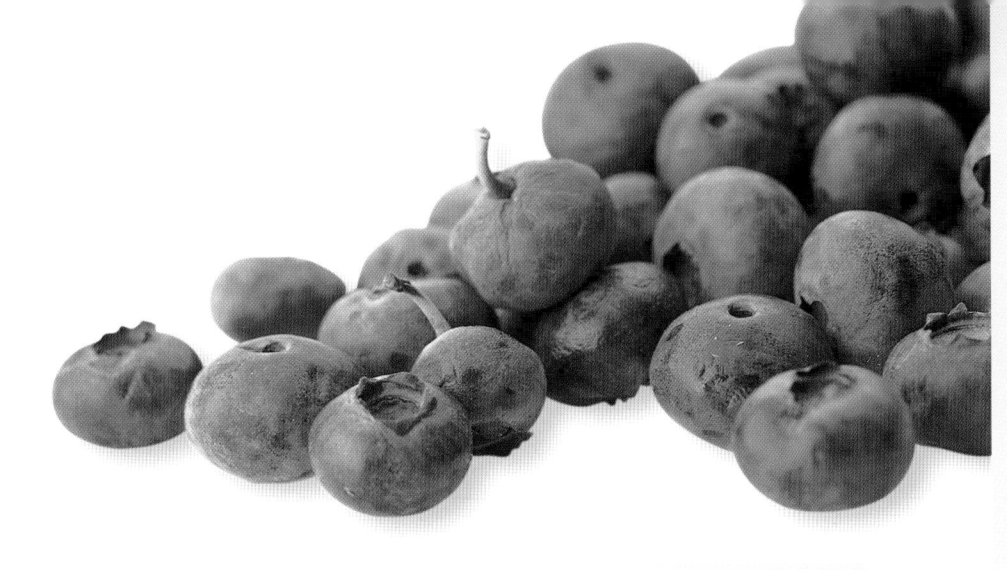

Blueberries

zzz

Originally popular mainly in the United States, blueberries are now enjoyed – and their nutritional value understood – worldwide. They are one of the richest sources of vitamin C, and may be eaten fresh, added to yoghurt or made into delicious muffins and pies.

calcium, magnesium, vitamin C

Cherries

zzz

This succulent fruit has a high level of vitamin C, required to convert tryptophan into serotonin, to ensure good-quality sleep. When not in season, the tinned variety may be used, as it tends to hold its vitamin C well, despite the processing.

calcium, magnesium, vitamin C

Halibut

zzzzzz

As an oily fish, halibut is rich in EFAs (omega-3) and contains calcium, chromium, copper, and vitamin B3. Excellent as a source of tryptophan from protein, all kinds of oily fish should be eaten regularly for dinner.

calcium, chromium, copper, omega-3 EFAs, tryptophan, vitamin B3

Kidney beans

zzz

One of the most abundant sources of calcium from a vegetarian source, kidney beans also provide beneficial fibre to help lower cholesterol and high blood pressure – factors that often contribute to sleep problems. They are also a good source of iron and B vitamins and, in addition, they have a low glycaemic index (that is, they release their sugars slowly), making them wonderful for balancing blood-sugar levels (see p.97).

calcium, iron, B vitamins

Tofu — zz

Derived from soya beans, tofu (bean curd) is considered another 'superfood', as it is a rich source of vegetarian protein, containing abundant vitamin B5; it also contains iron. It can be added to stir-fries, soups and casseroles, or blended in smoothies with fruit for a delicious night-time dessert.

iron, B vitamins

Barley — zzz

A good vegetarian source of both calcium and magnesium to encourage sleep, barley is also rich in the B-complex group of vitamins, which are required for balanced neurotransmission and sleep patterns. Added to soups and casseroles, barley makes a nutritious alternative to rice or potatoes.

calcium, magnesium, B vitamins

Yoghurt — zz

Plain bio-yoghurt (organic), which is unsweetened with sucrose or fructose, contains the amino acid tryptophan, needed for good-quality sleep. It is also a useful source of calcium, required for an efficient cardiovascular system. Adding plain yoghurt to fruit such as banana makes an excellent light pudding in the evening.

calcium, tryptophan

Almonds — zzzzzz

All nuts contain a balance of omega-3 and omega-6 EFAs (see p.76). Almonds also contain B vitamins and copper, abundant magnesium to balance their calcium, and they are a good vegetarian source of protein. They make a perfect late-night snack before retiring.

calcium, copper, magnesium, omega-3 and omega-6 EFAs, B vitamins

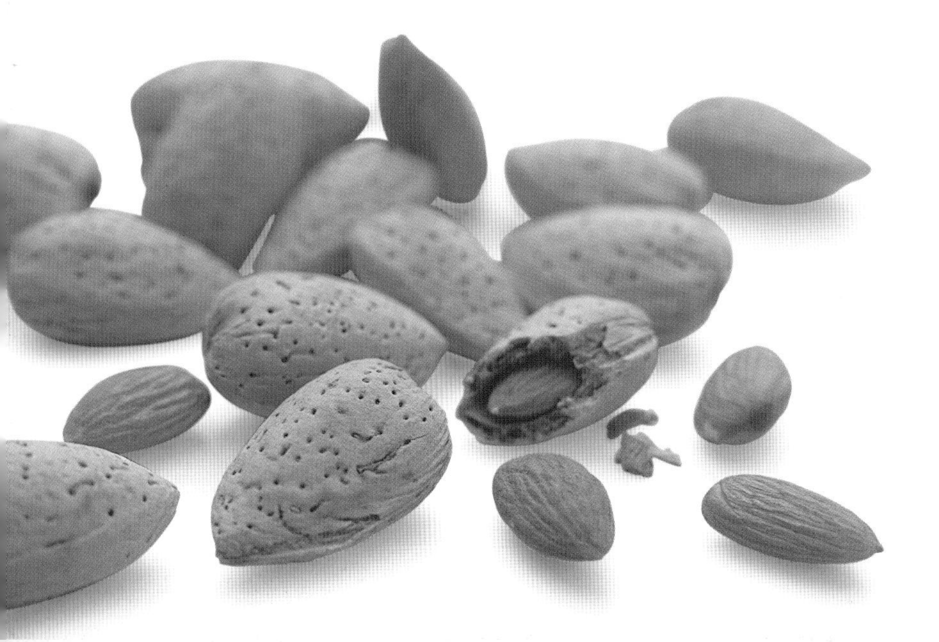

Eggs

zzzz

All eggs (hen, duck, goose, quail, ostrich, and so on) contain calcium and iron in their yolks and are a good source of vitamin B5. Being an animal protein, they are rich in tryptophan for encouraging sleep.

calcium, iron, tryptophan, B vitamins

Pak choi (or bok choy)

zzzz

Originally grown in the Orient, pak choi is now widely cultivated. It is one of the brassica family of vegetables, and thus contains abundant vitamin B5. Rich in both calcium and magnesium, this popular vegetable is a good choice for your evening meal.

calcium, magnesium, vitamins B and C

Mushrooms

zzzz

All types of mushrooms contain abundant B-complex vitamins, especially B5. Added to brown rice to make a risotto or to eggs for an omelette, mushrooms create a delicious evening meal to encourage relaxation and a sound night's sleep.

calcium, iron, magnesium, B vitamins

Peaches

zzzzz

Containing both calcium and magnesium, peaches are good for heart and cardiovascular health, helping to ensure that high blood pressure does not interfere with sleep patterns. They are also a rich source of vitamin C, which is required to convert tryptophan to serotonin, as well as helping the body manage stress – one of the main causes of insomnia.

calcium, copper, folic acid, magnesium, vitamin C

Walnuts zzzzzzz

All nuts are excellent sources of vegetarian protein, and walnuts have a particularly high content of the amino acid tryptophan, making them a good late-night snack, together with warm milk. Like other nuts, they are also a good source of calcium, copper, magnesium and B-complex vitamins.

calcium, copper, magnesium, omega-3 and omega-6 EFAs, tryptophan, B vitamins

Dates zzzz

A rich source of tryptophan is contained in this delicious fruit, which makes a good late-night snack, especially if combined with a small amount of natural bio-yoghurt.

calcium, iron, tryptophan, vitamin B3

Apricots zzzz

Another superb fruit for their mineral and vitamin content, apricots are rich in magnesium, iron and copper. They also contain plenty of vitamins B3 and B5, so they make a perfect pudding or late-night snack with some yoghurt or cream.

copper, iron, magnesium, B vitamins

Apples zzz

The humble apple will always feature on a sleep-well programme, as it contains a beneficial balance of calcium and magnesium, if the whole fruit (including the skin) is consumed. As a good source of fibre, apples encourage sound blood-sugar management; they also contain vitamin C.

calcium, magnesium, vitamin C

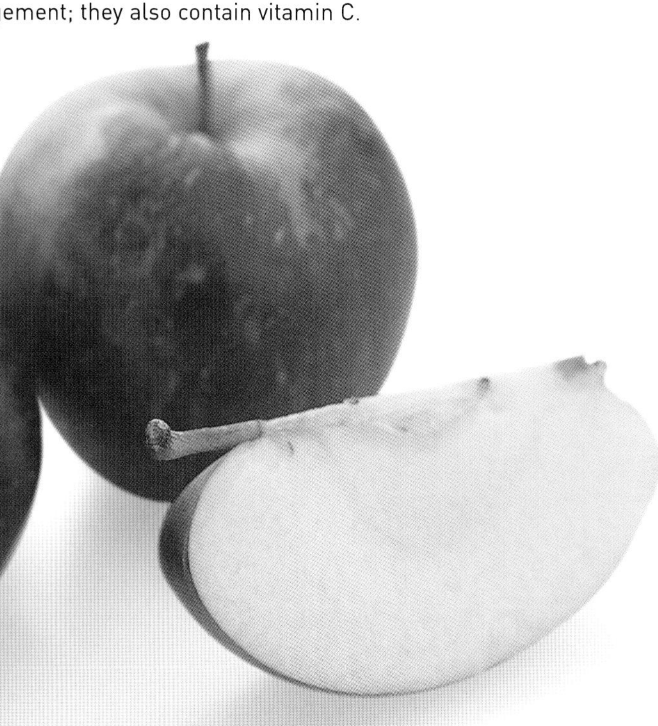

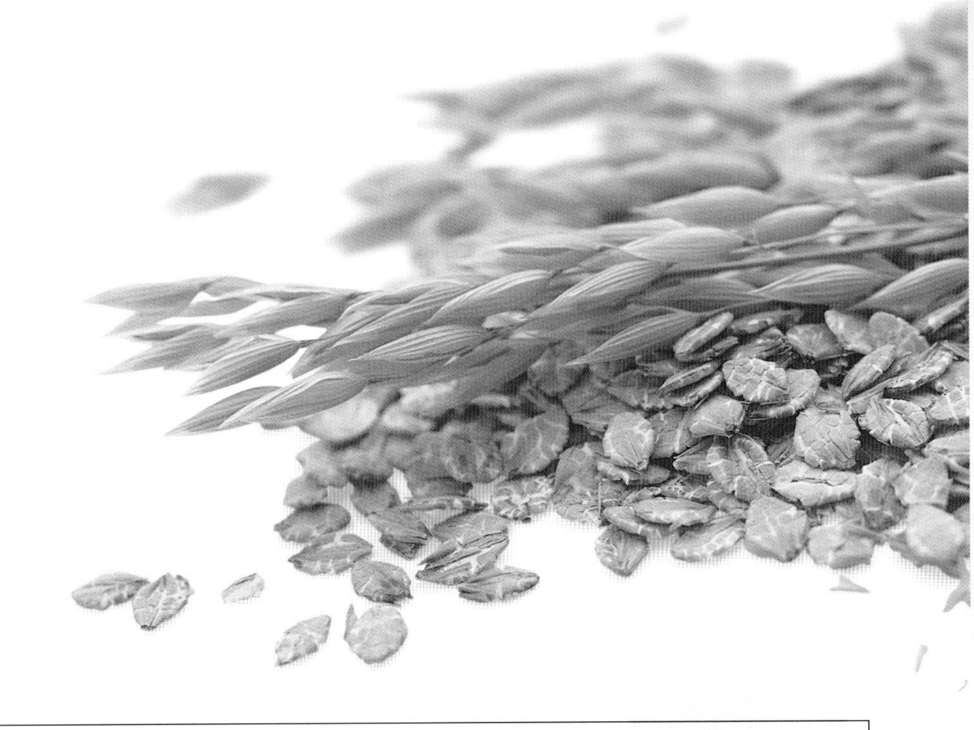

Oats **zzzzz**

Rich in B-complex vitamins – as are all grains – oats are an excellent source of copper. As a beneficial source of fibre, they help to regulate blood pressure and encourage good blood-sugar management. They are also a good source of calcium, iron and magnesium.

calcium, copper, iron, magnesium, B vitamins

Cottage cheese **zzz**

As a low-fat cheese, this is known for its high levels of tryptophan, and can therefore be eaten in the evening without the worry of overburdening the digestive system. Eaten on its own, or with apricots or figs for their magnesium content, cottage cheese makes a good choice for the end of the meal.

calcium, tryptophan, B vitamins

Asparagus **zzzz**

Rich in B vitamins to relax the mind after a busy day, asparagus also contains a compound called inulin, which has insulin-like properties to encourage good blood-sugar management (see p.97). It makes an ideal light supper served on its own or as an addition to a salad.

calcium, magnesium, vitamins B and C

Millet **zzz**

A lesser-known grain, millet has a low glycaemic index (required for balancing blood-sugar levels, see page 98), and is a rich source of both magnesium and potassium, which is associated with heart and cardiovascular health, as well as with regulating cellular exchanges of nutrients and toxins. Millet flakes make an excellent alternative to oats for a fruit crumble.

magnesium, potassium, vitamin B3

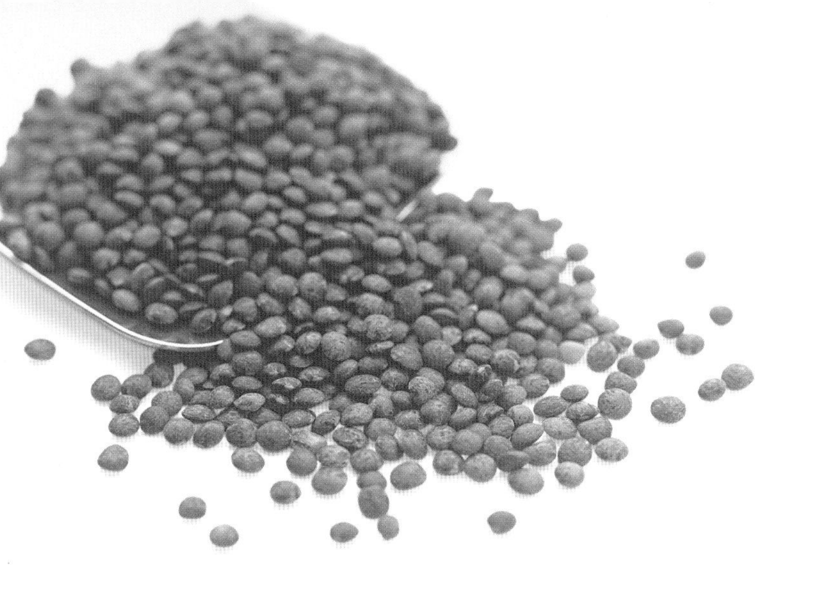

Lentils

zzz

copper, iron, B vitamins

Lentils are one of the most nutritious vegetarian sources of protein as well as an excellent source of iron, copper and the B group of vitamins. They are particularly high in vitamin B5 (pantothenic acid), which is required by the adrenal glands to manage stress and create relaxation. Not all lentils need soaking before cooking, and may be used on their own or as part of the Indian dish dhal.

Sunflower seeds

zzzz

calcium, omega-3 and omega-6 EFAs, B vitamins

Containing good levels of omega-3 and omega-6 EFAs, these little seeds are also a beneficial source of calcium and B vitamins, making them a perfect addition to salads, soups and puddings with the evening meal to encourage a good night's sleep.

Potatoes

zzzzz

calcium, copper, magnesium, vitamins B3 and C

The humble potato should never be excluded from a list of healthy foods, as it is rich in vitamin C as well as copper. B vitamins also abound in potatoes, which are highly versatile in the ways in which they may be cooked.

Raisins

zzzz

calcium, folic acid, iron, magnesium

Raisins are one of the highest fruit sources of iron, although they are also high in fruit sugars, so they should be eaten with grains and protein to balance blood-sugar management (see p.97). They are a perfect addition to breakfast cereal, and the absorption and utilization of their minerals in the body takes several hours, so the benefits are derived at night-time.

z Each z represents a sleepy nutrient.

Sardines

zzz

As well as being a rich source of omega-3 EFAs, sardines have high levels of calcium for regulating the cycles of sleep as well as the heartbeat. They are perfect with rye toast for a light evening meal.

calcium, chromium, omega-3 EFAs

Buckwheat

zzzzz

Being a member of the rhubarb family, buckwheat is not strictly a wheat and is the one grain that contains all eight essential amino acids that are usually found only in animal protein. Also rich in calcium and magnesium, it encourages good sleep. Buckwheat noodles make an excellent alternative to wheat-flour pasta, and buckwheat itself is frequently used in soup dishes in Oriental cooking.

calcium, magnesium, omega-6 EFAs, tryptophan, vitamin C

Bananas

zzzzz

One of the richest fruit sources of tryptophan, bananas have for centuries been part of an old wives' tale for beating insomnia (see p.106). Teamed with strawberries for their vitamin C, they make the perfect sleep-inducing evening pudding, or may be eaten on their own in the middle of the night to combat insomnia. Bananas are also rich sources of copper and magnesium.

copper, magnesium, tryptophan, vitamins B6 and C

Pineapples

zzzz

Known to contain a high level of tryptophan, pineapple is a good source of the vitamin C required to convert tryptophan into serotonin, to ensure a good night's sleep. Add to yoghurt for a delicious pudding at dinner.

calcium, magnesium, tryptophan, vitamin C

lazy weekend

FOOD PLAN

FRIDAY NIGHT

For supper have some **Bean Soup with Spring Greens** (see p.132). Alternatively, you can use bought fresh organic vegetable soup – preferably one that includes green vegetables (such as watercress, broccoli, parsley and spinach), as these are rich in magnesium, which is required to promote relaxation and a good night's sleep. Treat yourself to a couple of squares of dark chocolate (preferably at least 80 per cent cocoa content), as it is a delicious source of minerals (but ensure that its sugar content is as low as possible, as refined sugar can influence magnesium levels and disturb sleep).

SATURDAY

Breakfast

Eat some fresh fruit salad that includes oranges, strawberries, kiwi fruit and blueberries, all of which are excellent sources of vitamin C (see p. 76). Add two or three tablespoons of live bio-yoghurt and sprinkle liberally with linseeds (for their protein content).

Mid-morning snack

Have a herbal tea with toasted rye bread or pumpernickel, spread with half a ripe avocado, to provide essential fats and fibre. Avocados are perfect snack foods, as they contain the ideal balance of protein, carbohydrates and EFAs.

Lunch

Serve some fresh poached salmon, served with a selection of salad leaves and a few raw vegetables from your shopping basket, to ensure a nutritious lunch that will provide the perfect balance between food groups. This is also an easy dish to prepare with minimum fuss. Eat an apple afterwards to clear the palate and aid digestion.

Here is a plan for a lazy weekend, designed to enhance your slumber and reduce your stress levels, leaving you feeling rested and refreshed. In preparation for the weekend, reduce your consumption of regular tea, coffee and other caffeinated drinks, such as colas, from the middle of the week. If possible, plan to visit your supermarket or food store on Thursday so that you can stock up on the essentials for the weekend (see the shopping list on p.90) .

Mid-afternoon snack

Feel free to indulge in a selection of fresh fruit, such as plums, grapes and apricots, all of which are rich in vitamins and minerals to encourage the elimination of the week's bad eating habits and stresses.

Dinner

Minimize your cooking by preparing a one-pot meal. Take a fresh chicken and make the **Lazy Chicken Pot recipe** (see p.136). While the chicken is cooking, soak in a warm bath, perhaps adding some essential oils to enhance relaxation. After dinner, retire as early as possible, eating a banana just before you go to bed to encourage sleep.

SUNDAY

Breakfast/brunch

When you wake, make a pot of chamomile tea to take back to bed with you, preferably with the Sunday papers!

Later in the morning prepare a brunch of smoked salmon and eggs with some toasted rye bread or pumpernickel – a high-protein meal that should provide you with enough energy to last through the afternoon.

Mid-afternoon snack

Crudités and hummus make an excellent snack requiring very little preparation, and help to take the edge off your hunger and discourage unhealthy snacking.

Evening meal

You should have some chicken left over from last night, the flavour of which will be even better today, so prepare a plate of cold chicken with steamed vegetables. Drizzle with a little **Herb Dressing** (see p.135) and top with sesame seeds for flavour.

SHOPPING LIST

You need to buy enough fresh produce to see you through until breakfast on Monday, so that you do not have to interrupt your lazy weekend with food shopping. If the suggested produce is out of season, choose other seasonal fruits or vegetables – the important factor here is variety and freshness. The quantities given below are for two people.

You will also need to add the ingredients for the following recipes to your shopping list.

Bean Soup with Spring Greens (see p.132)
Lazy Chicken Pot (see p.136)
Herb Dressing (see p.135)

4 oranges
2 punnets of strawberries
4 kiwi fruit
2 punnets of blueberries
tub of live bio-yoghurt
packet of linseeds or sesame seeds
2–3 boxes of herbal teas (see p.91 for suggestions)
loaf of rye bread or pumpernickel
2 avocados
4oz/125g fresh poached salmon
1lb/500g assorted salad leaves
6 apples or pears
4 red plums
medium-sized bunch of grapes
4 apricots
selection of fresh herbs
4 bananas
1lb/500g smoked salmon
2 eggs
tub of hummus
1 small jar mustard
1 small packet sesame seeds
10½pt/6 litres of mineral water
small bar of dark chocolate

ESSENTIAL TIPS

1 Make no plans at all – this is your time off.
2 Switch off your telephones and do not check your e-mails.
3 Ensure that you have plenty of reading material.
4 Eat when you feel hungry, not according to the clock.
5 Eat early in the evening to allow your digestive system to calm down before you sleep.

Drinks

Avoid excessive amounts of alcohol, as it interferes with sleep.
Reduce or omit coffee and tea (other than herbal – see below), as these are stimulating and stressful to the body in general.
Increase your intake of mineral water, drinking 4½–5pt/2.5–3 litres daily (including herbal teas).

Herbal teas

Chamomile – relaxes the body and induces sleepiness
Nettle – a natural diuretic and good for eliminating toxins
Fennel – cleansing and refreshing
Rosehip and orange – high in vitamin C and raises immunity
Ginger and lemon – a good pick-me-up in the morning

Essential oils

Essential oils can be used in a variety of ways to calm the mind and body – in the bath, in a vaporizer or by putting just a few drops of neat oil on your pillow to soothe you as you fall asleep. Never use essential oils neat on the skin, as they must be combined with a base oil such as almond. Different herbs have different qualities – some herbs are energizing, but the following all have soothing qualities:

Geranium – relaxing for the mind and muscles
Lavender – encourages deep sleep
Neroli – healing and sleep-inducing
Thyme – restorative and relaxing

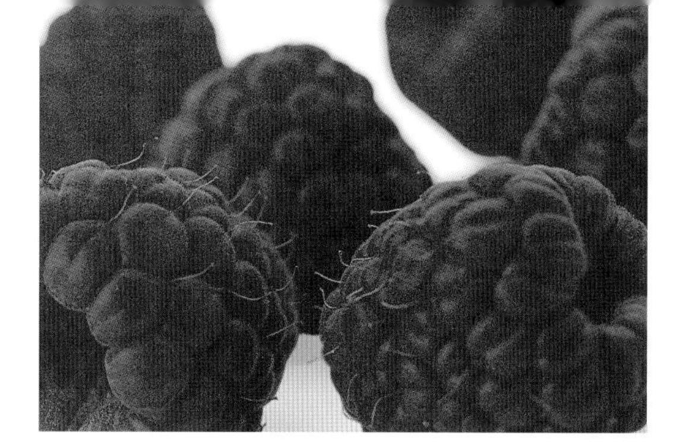

what

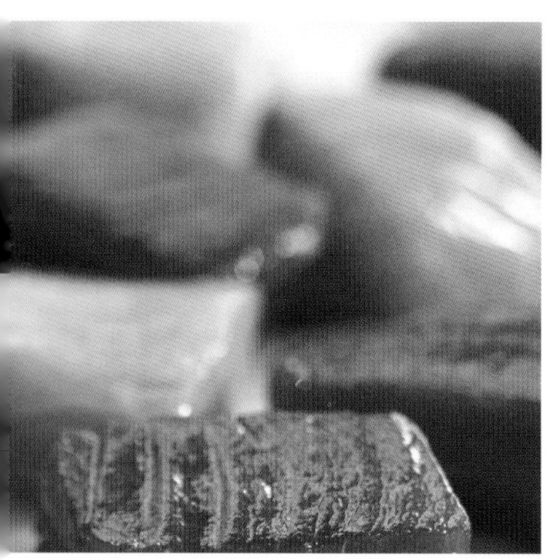

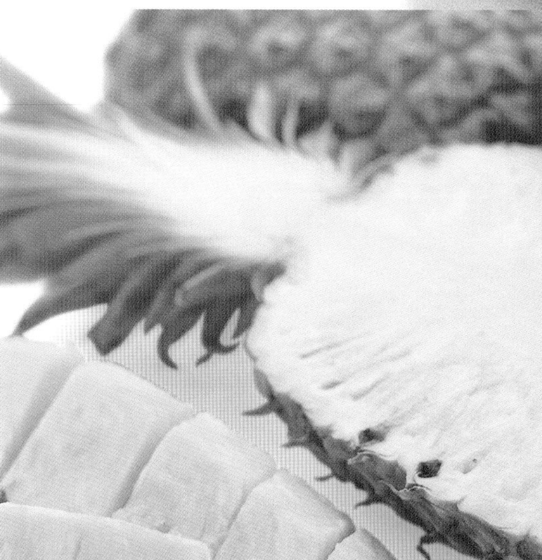

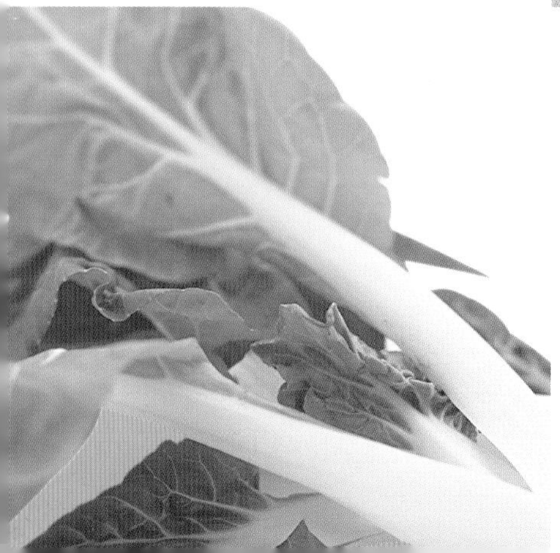

can affect your sleep?

factors which affect your ability to have a good night's sleep

There are many contributing factors to disrupted sleep patterns, some of which are external and beyond our control, whilst others originate from the internal workings of our bodies.

We have already looked in depth at how stress affects our libido (see pages 54–55 and 59–63), and the same can be said of our sleep – a busy mind prevents us from falling asleep and may interfere with the normal five-part process to our sleep patterns. Allowing time to unwind at the end of the day is critical to inducing deep sleep.

What we eat can have a profound effect on our ability to get to, and remain, asleep. Heavy or spicy meals are stimulating and a burden to the digestive system, which works at its best earlier in the day. Choose lighter meals in the evening, particularly if you are eating late, and don't go to bed for at least an hour after finishing your meal. Blood-sugar management is key to promoting deep and restorative sleep, as we shall see further on.

Remember that stimulants, such as tea, coffee and alcohol, disrupt blood-sugar management, so these drinks should be kept to a minimum to ensure a good night's sleep.

problems

In order to explore the problems associated with sleep, it is important to understand how our body's cycle works on a day-to-day basis. We can then look at how this cycle becomes disrupted and at what major contributing factors affect our precious sleep.

circadian rhythms

Each person functions best on a different number of hours sleep per day, but it is not simply an old wives' tale that each hour spent asleep before midnight is worth two hours for each one after midnight. The body responds to what is known as the circadian rhythm – the 24-hour biological clock during which each hour holds a special time for each major organ of the body.

The following chart indicates the optimal functioning time of each major body organ. It is interesting to note that the gall bladder, liver and lung functions are at their optimum while we sleep – the liver and gall bladder being the organs of detoxification of all ingested foods, drinks and medication, of hormone regulation and of cholesterol production/balance; and the lungs the proprietors of oxygen regulation. The large intestine – being the last organ in the digestive tract – works optimally to clear itself when the least amount of food is being ingested. This is not to say that these organs do not function well at other times of the day; simply that the importance of sleep should not be underestimated in terms of our body's ability to restore and rebalance itself.

CIRCADIAN CLOCK

1 a.m.–3 a.m.	liver	1 p.m.–3 p.m.	small intestine
3 a.m.–5 a.m.	lung	3 p.m.–5 p.m.	bladder
5 a.m.–7 a.m.	large intestine	5 p.m.–7 p.m.	kidney
7 a.m.–9 a.m.	stomach	7 p.m.–9 p.m.	circulation/sexual function
9 a.m.–11 a.m.	spleen	9 p.m.–11 p.m.	thyroid function
11 a.m.–1p.m.	heart	11 p.m.–1 a.m.	gall bladder

Marvellous melatonin

The circadian rhythm is regulated by a hormone released from the pineal gland at the base of the skull, called melatonin. Much has been researched and written on this fascinating hormone over the last ten years, as it is said to hold the secrets to anti-ageing, relieving depression, aiding immunity (as a powerful antioxidant) and redressing the problems associated with jetlag (see below). Melatonin is itself derived from another hormone, called serotonin, which controls nerve transmission in the brain, regulating mood and states of consciousness, and is sometimes known as the 'happy hormone'. Those suffering from depression may have low levels of serotonin, and this can consequently interfere with sleep patterns and sufficiency. Increasing melatonin levels may be induced by regulating serotonin, and as tryptophan is the precursor to serotonin you should increase your intake of tryptophan-rich foods (see p.106).

The human sleep pattern works on a diurnal basis – that is, it is affected by night and day, and we are naturally most active during the hours of light. Our production of melatonin rises gradually from the setting of the sun (or loss of natural light) and recedes at the onset of morning light.

JET LAG

Jetlag occurs as the body becomes confused by its reception of outside stimuli, namely sunlight, as time zones are traversed more rapidly than would normally occur during a 24-hour day (or even in reverse). If we travel frequently, particularly across several time zones, our circadian rhythm is thrown out of balance and takes several days to recover. One of the most important aids to this vital function is water – dehydration is one of the main causes of jetlag, but water gives us the ability to rebalance the body after long-haul flights.

International flying is now commonplace, yet it is interesting to note that pilots, stewards and stewardesses have the highest level of insomnia problems (see p.98), as well as hormonal disruptions, which can affect their fertility and upset their digestive systems. When we look at the organ functions of the circadian rhythm, this becomes easier to understand.

stress

As we have seen in relation to sex (p.44), stress triggers a number of hormonal responses. If we consider the effects that these stress-induced hormones have on the body, then it is easy to see how stress can interrupt sleep patterns.

When adrenaline is released from the adrenal glands in response to stress, it raises the heart rate, slows digestion and encourages the release of glycogen (stored glucose) from the muscles and liver. If adrenaline is stimulated late in the evening, this is likely to prevent you from falling asleep.

Many situations can induce stress, and avoiding those pressures that you know to be stressful can obviously help improve sleep patterns, although this may not always be practical. The first step is to identify your potential sources of stress.

Food allergies and intolerances

One potential source of internal stress is the food that we eat. If you have an allergy which involves a rapid response to a food or type of food, or have developed an intolerance (a milder response, producing symptoms up to three days after consumption), then this will trigger the release of adrenaline. Subsequent increased heart rate and alertness inhibit falling asleep and may be involved in keeping you awake long after you intended.

If you have an undiagnosed food intolerance to, say, wheat, then every time you eat pasta, bread or any other food that contains wheat or wheat flour, adrenaline will be released. If you eat a typical evening meal that includes bread or pasta, then adrenaline is likely to keep you awake late into the evening. This might be quite welcome if you are not feeling tired, but it is quite likely that the undiagnosed intolerance will have been involved in interrupting your sleep patterns for some time.

Food allergies are, thankfully, quite rare, and although one US survey reported that 40 per cent of those asked felt that they had a food allergy, the true figure is actually nearer 2 per cent. It is food intolerances that are far more prevalent. These are often hard to diagnose and pinpoint, due to a diverse range of symptoms, most of which are never even associated with food. If someone with an intolerance to wheat were to eat that same evening meal, then the reaction would be far milder, but would probably affect sleep in the early part of the night, since the stress reaction would be less intense than it would be for an allergy.

Identifying food intolerances and allergies is therefore an important step to take in improving sleep patterns. The most common allergens are wheat, citrus fruit, dairy foods and nuts; wheat and dairy products are again the most likely causes of food intolerances. Perversely, it is often a food that we feel drawn to, or eat most frequently, that may be involved in reducing our sleep time. So try to be aware of your intake of the most likely culprits, and work with a qualified nutritional consultant to identify those foods that may be contributing to your health issues. Do be aware that food-allergy tests are rarely fully accurate, and often identify foods as potential problems that are in fact simply the foods that were eaten most recently. Beware of expensive tests that are not carried out under the auspices of an appropriate professional.

The most common allergens are wheat, citrus fruit, dairy foods and nuts.

Cortisol and sleep

Cortisol is another hormone released by the adrenal gland at times of stress, or (in the long term) after a prolonged period of stress. Cortisol enhances the body's utilization of fats, carbohydrates and especially protein, increasing glucose production. This has the effect of increasing blood-sugar levels (see p.97), making the individual feel alert and awake. If cortisol is released late at night, then it is very likely to inhibit sleep, as the body will not be in a natural state of relaxation, but rather in a state of excitation. This can occur even if the individual is feeling fatigued and longing for sleep. Repeated stimulation of the adrenal glands can lead to adrenal insufficiency or exhaustion. This condition is common in people who are 'high fliers' – the small amount of sleep that they seem to need is often admired, yet their lack of sleep will have many repercussions on their health and abilities.

As with adrenaline, avoiding stressful situations and identifying food intolerances or allergies is of primary importance in reducing cortisol production. Cortisol is also produced during strenuous exercise, so playing a sport in the evenings (even directly after work) may be linked to sleeping problems. Note whether your sleep patterns improve on the days that you do not engage in your chosen sport. If you do notice benefits, then consider changing your habits to exercise at other times of the day, as sleep is just as important to the body as exercise.

blood-sugar management

Much of the food that we eat is converted into glucose (see p.98), which circulates in the body, supplying fuel to every cell, which is in turn used to create energy. The levels of glucose in the blood fluctuate almost constantly, as energy expenditure increases and decreases. When blood-sugar levels are low, stored glucose (glycogen) is released from the muscles and liver to maintain equilibrium, and more food is required to sustain glucose production. We experience this as hunger.

How long we can go without eating differs in each of us, and is dependent on several factors. If food, or fuel, is lacking, then the body must force the muscles and liver to release more of its glycogen, and it is this mechanism that can interrupt our sleep patterns and is often one of the contributory factors to waking in the small hours.

How to prevent fluctuations

When we are asleep our energy requirements are naturally lower than they are when we are awake. But the brain is still working, and since it is the largest single user of glucose, if glucose levels drop, then they must be replenished immediately; however, as we are asleep, eating is not an option. If the glucose levels required exceed those that can be released at normal speed from the liver and muscles, then the body has to find a way to increase glycogen release. Although this is as yet unproven, it seems logical that this involves the hormones adrenaline and cortisol. As we have seen (p.95), adrenaline increases both heart rate and alertness, and thus we awaken with a thumping heart, suddenly feeling wide-awake, but unrefreshed. This scenario is especially prevalent after drinking alcohol during the evening. Alcohol is a simple sugar, which raises blood-sugar levels quickly, resulting in a sharper than usual drop during the night. The same effect is often noticed when a high-sugar food is eaten late in the evening.

If this sounds familiar, then avoiding alcohol in the evenings is essential, as is consuming excess refined sugar. Eating a little protein and fibre before retiring can also help, even if this is just a mouthful of cottage cheese and half an apple, which slow down glucose release.

THE GLYCAEMIC INDEX

The speed at which foods are broken down by the digestive tract differs enormously, with some being converted into glucose rapidly, while other foods are slower to digest. Glucose levels in the blood fluctuate constantly and are influenced by which foods we choose to eat.

Those foods that are converted into glucose quickly have a high value in what is known as the glycaemic index (GI). This is a table that charts the rate of energy release of everyday foods. Simple carbohydrates tend to have a high GI, while proteins and complex carbohydrates usually have a lower GI, as they take longer to digest and break down.

If simple carbohydrates (with a high GI) are eaten on their own, they can cause a surge in blood-sugar levels, leading to high insulin levels. This can in turn lead to excess body fat and to lows in energy levels. To avoid these highs and subsequent lows, you should eat foods with a lower GI, or combine high-GI foods with low-scoring foods. The rule of the thumb is that the sweeter the food, the higher its GI.

For example, butter beans score 32, while a rice cake scores 81; beetroot (beet) scores 64 and parsnip 97. If you were to eat a rice cake on its own, then it would probably cause an eventual low, but eating an apple (with a GI of 37) in the same snack would mean that the average GI was 81 + 37 ÷ 2 = 59.

By choosing foods with a medium to low GI, it is more likely that your blood-sugar levels will stay balanced and that your energy levels will be more consistent.

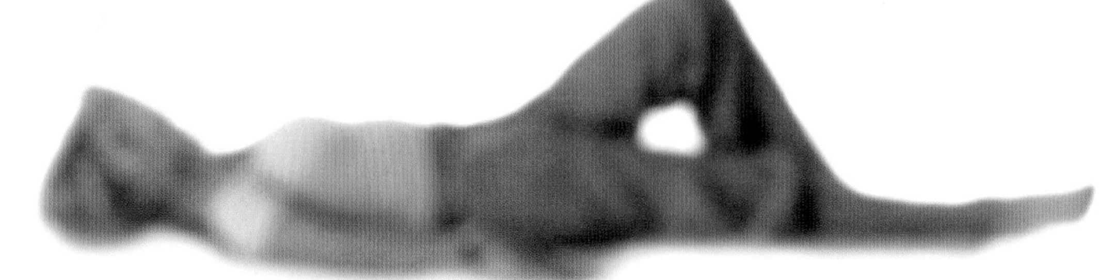

insomnia

There is no ideal amount of sleep for which we should be aiming. Our biochemical individuality means that four hours sleep is enough for some people, while others require at least eight hours. On average, we spend as much as 35 per cent of our lives asleep, and a lack of sleep can cause any number of problems. Yet despite endless research, scientists are still not agreed on the causes of disrupted sleep patterns. One of the most common conditions, insomnia, is thought to affect 20 per cent of the western population, yet almost 75 per cent claim to have experienced insomnia at one time or another. Insomnia is a continued lack of sleep that leaves the individual feeling fatigued most of the time. Not being able to fall asleep, waking at intervals throughout the night or waking early in the morning and being unable to get back to sleep are all symptoms of insomnia.

Insomnia falls into two main types. The first, known as occasional or transient insomnia, is the most prevalent. As the name suggests, it is a short-term condition, sometimes associated with events in our lives. It may last for a few nights or for as long as a few weeks.

Chronic insomnia, on the other hand, is a condition that can deprive the individual of adequate sleep for months, years or, in extreme cases, for an entire lifetime.

Anxiety and tension

Both of these are likely to be a factor in short-term insomnia. In the long term, however, a lifetime of stress can disrupt the action of the adrenal glands, which in turn leads to either an overproduction of adrenaline or possibly to adrenaline being produced in the middle of the night, causing the individual to wake with a pounding heart (see p.95). Try having a small snack, designed to help balance blood-sugar levels (see p.97), before going to bed to counteract the short-term effects of anxiety; more importantly, try to resolve the causes of tension in the first place.

Anyone with sleep problems should avoid caffeine altogether, or at least limit their intake to one cup of tea or coffee in the early part of the day.

Depression

One of the most common symptoms of clinical depression is insomnia. This lack of sleep can easily exacerbate feelings of depression, and many doctors prescribe a type of anti-depressant drug known as a 'tricyclic anti-depressant'. This is also often prescribed for people suffering from insomnia but not from depression, as it works to calm the central nervous system (CNS), which is thought to promote sleep, yet the doses are not high enough to affect the mood of the individual. Despite relatively low doses, dependency can occur, and the root cause of the insomnia may never be discovered. In addition, nearly all anti-depressants can interfere with the REM stage of sleep (see p.66), so that when we wake in the morning we may still feel tired because the deepest phase of sleep has been missed.

Depression is often linked to low serotonin levels, and modern anti-depressants work directly on increasing levels of serotonin in the brain. This has the effect of lifting mood and promoting more regular sleep patterns. To boost your serotonin levels, increase your intake of tryptophan-rich foods (see p.106).

Stimulants

Caffeine is known to stimulate the CNS and thus inhibit sleep. Many people find that they become more sensitive to caffeine as they age and just one cup of coffee or tea (since regular tea also contains caffeine) can keep them awake for hours. Many insomniacs therefore avoid caffeine in the latter part of the day. We would advise anyone with sleep problems (especially insomnia) to avoid caffeine altogether, or at least to limit their intake to one cup of tea or coffee in the early part of the day.

Decaffeinated coffee is not always the answer, as coffee acts as a diuretic and, although you may drift off to sleep naturally, the urge to urinate may wake you up repeatedly through the night. And do remember that caffeine is found not just in tea and coffee, but in many carbonated drinks (even 'diet' or 'lite' versions), chocolate drinks and over-the-counter medicines for colds.

Food intake

The digestive system works throughout the night, albeit at a lower rate than during waking hours. If your evening meal is excessive – either in size or in terms of sugars and fats – then the digestive system has to work at an increased rate to cope. If you suffer from insomnia, eating lightly in the evening could help promote prolonged sleep. Your evening meal should be completed at least two hours before you intend to sleep and should include a little protein, fibre and carbohydrate for maximum blood-sugar management. Some foods are known to have an excitatory or stimulating effect on the CNS and should be excluded whenever possible. This includes highly spiced food that contains chillies or large amounts of garlic or ginger.

Dieting

Many overweight people have trouble sleeping, and this may be due in no small part to their cycles of dieting and eating. If you have experienced insomnia and are a regular dieter, then it may be your low calorie intake that is affecting your sleep quality. Bear in mind that there are several reasons why we lose or gain weight, and what we eat is just one factor. Weight management is inextricably connected to good health, so it may be worth investigating other areas of your health and improving your overall status, without making weight loss your sole goal.

People on a low-calorie diet often wake during the night, which may in part be due to fluctuating or low blood-sugar levels (see p.97). Remember that the digestive system carries on working through the night and, as the liver's optimum functioning time is 1–3 a.m. (see p.94), stored glucose may be released then from the liver, as glycogen, to meet the body's demands for energy production to carry out the rebuilding processes that occur during the night. This in turn induces the possibility of waking in the middle of the night and feeling wide awake, with the frustration of not being able to go back to sleep. Try the blood-sugar balance snacks on p.101 to counteract this.

AVOIDING TYRAMINE

Foods that contain the amino acid tyramine are thought to increase the production of a substance known as noradrenaline (norepinephrine in the United States). This is known to inhibit the sleep process, although perversely noradrenaline is required in small amounts for effective REM sleep stages (see p.66). However, it is best not to encourage the production of noradrenaline, so avoiding tyramine-rich foods is advisable. These include sugar, chocolate, sauerkraut, bacon, ham, sausage, cheese, aubergines (eggplants), potatoes, tomatoes, peppers and smoked meats and fish.

Age

Many older people sleep for fewer hours than they did in their younger days. A 1997 survey of British teenagers and pensioners highlighted some fascinating traits. Teenagers are renowned for sleeping late, yet they often complain of feeling tired – in the survey they reported that they required at least eight hours of sleep a night, but still often felt fatigued. However, the over-65s who were questioned reported that they needed less sleep (usually five to six hours a night), and thought that their sleep was of a better quality as they felt refreshed when they woke. The reasons for this are not fully understood. It could be as simple as needing less sleep as we get older, or more intricately linked to circadian rhythms (see p.94) that alter with time. Whatever group you fall into, following some simple nutrition and lifestyle tips (see below) should help to combat insomnia.

LIFESTYLE TIPS FOR COMBATING INSOMNIA

In addition to improving your nutritional status, there are changes in routine and lifestyle that can help you normalize your sleep patterns:

1. If you cannot sleep, do not linger in bed waiting for sleep to occur. Get out of bed, read a book or listen to some quiet, relaxing music. Return to bed when you feel ready to sleep.
2. Do not watch the clock, as this can increase your anxiety over lack of sleep.
3. Promote relaxation wherever possible, perhaps with long walks or warm (but not too hot) baths in the evening.
4. Avoid stressful situations in the evening, and learn how to prepare for sleep gently and without stress.
5. Avoid watching violent or potentially upsetting television or video films immediately prior to retiring. Once stimulated, the brain takes a considerable time to calm down, which is bound to interfere with your quality of sleep.

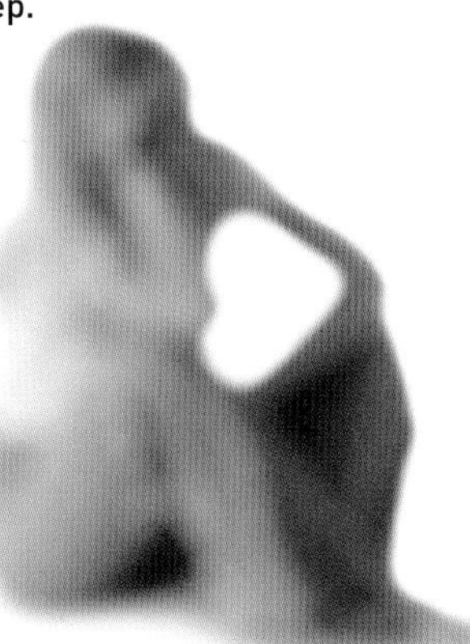

IDEAL SLEEP SNACKS

- Banana and soya-milk smoothie
- Plain yoghurt with chopped dates
- Low-fat cottage cheese with oat cakes
- Mixed sunflower and sesame seeds with apple slices
- Rye bread with slices of turkey

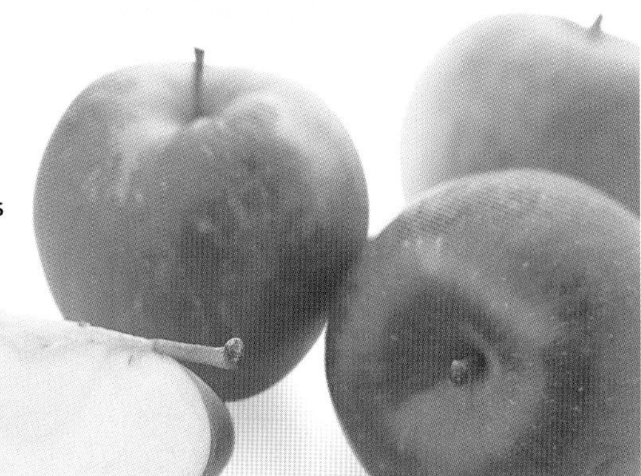

sleep problems

Sleep problems such as snoring may seem to be trivial at first, but they can quickly become very debilitating and start to take on huge significance in your life. Diet may well be a factor, but serious conditions such as apnoea and narcolepsy may require lifestyle changes and/or medical intervention.

SNORING

It is long-standing joke (for all those who don't sleep with a snoring partner!) that snoring will interrupt the sleep of even the heaviest sleepers, but why does snoring happen to some people and not others? There are a number of reasons why people snore, some of which are physical, although most of them originate from dietary or lifestyle choices.

From a physical point of view, the size, shape and structure of the nose may be the main contributory factor to snoring. There may be a structural obstruction, such as a deviated septum (the partition between the two sides of the nose), or a group of polyps that have obstructed the air passage. During the day such people will breathe through their mouths, but during sleep they lose this choice, resulting in a struggle to get sufficient air to the lungs.

During sleep, the soft palate (the fleshy portion of the roof of the mouth) and the tongue relax. In some people this may cause a compression of the throat, leading to vibrations that result in snoring. Those who tend to lie on their back while sleeping generally snore more than those who lie on their side, as this physical effect is emphasized in the flat-on-the-back position. This is the main reason for encouraging a snorer to turn over onto his or her side during sleep.

Smoking and alcohol consumption are two of the main factors that contribute to snoring, as they interfere with the minute cilia (fine hairs) that line the nasal passage, and with the bronchioles (tubes leading to the air sacs) of the lungs. Both indulgences inhibit absorption of the nutrients that are essential for relaxing and restful sleep, and even passive smoking (non-smokers being exposed to cigarette fumes in public places) can increase the likelihood of snoring.

Mild food intolerances may also be at the root of a snoring problem, and it is worth considering what you have consumed during the day when the problem occurs – any food that causes inflammation of the digestive tissues (from the mouth downwards) could restrict the air passages. Keep a 'snore and snack' food diary to monitor possible culprits, noting the particular foods eaten every day; if the problem occurs repeatedly, you may then be able to identify foods that are common to several snoring incidents. You can eliminate certain foods from your diet on a trial basis, but long-term removal should only be done on the advice of a nutritional consultant or doctor to ensure correct nutritional balance.

Dairy products are known to be mucus-forming and can considerably exacerbate mild snoring, by partially blocking the airways to the lungs. Changing over to alternatives to dairy foods made from cow's milk, including oat-milk, rice-milk and soya-milk products, has proven in many cases of

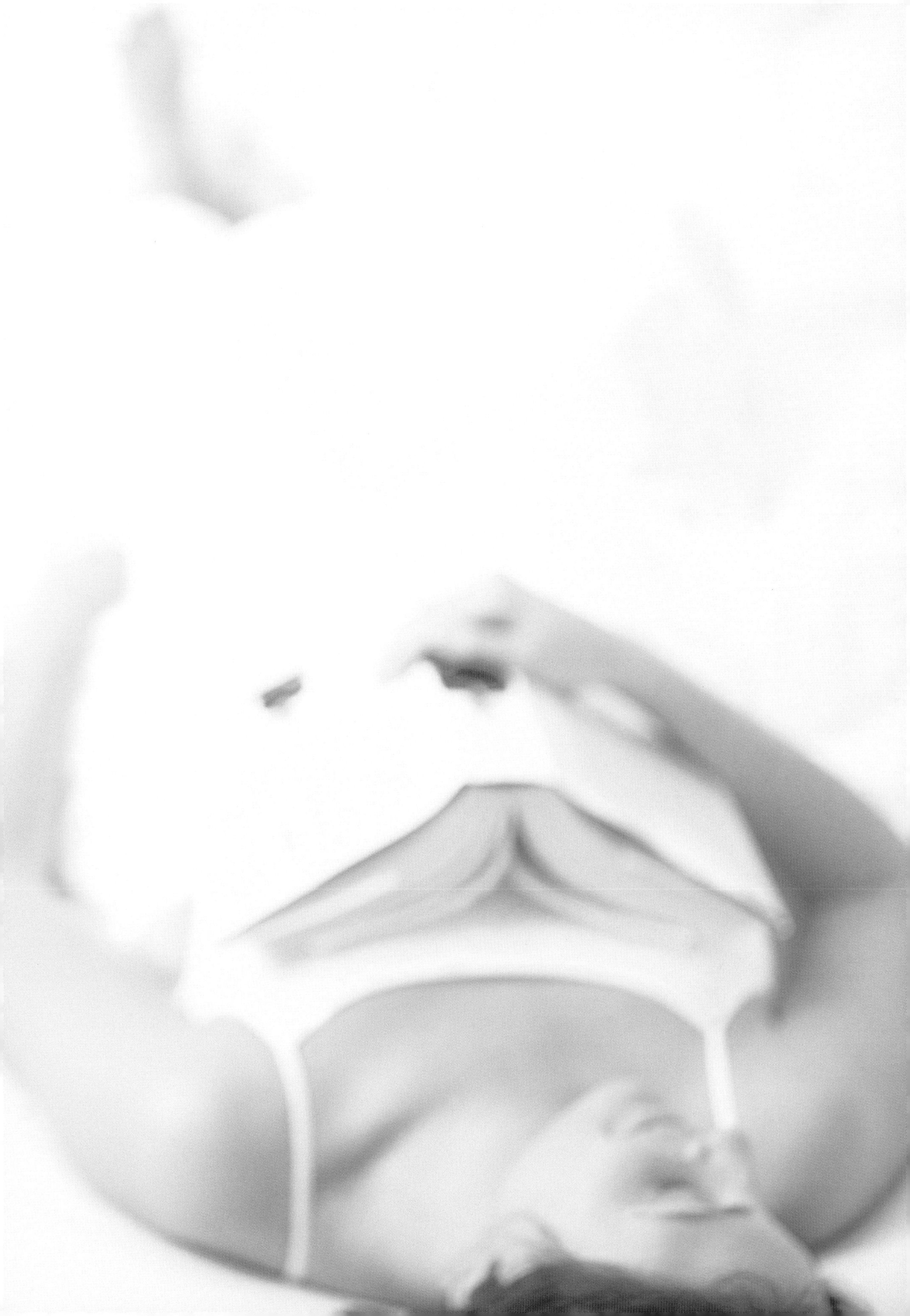

snoring that dairy foods were the sole contributory factor. Eliminating cow's milk and other dairy products for as little as two weeks may change the annoying habit of a lifetime! Severe cases of snoring may be associated with sleep apnoea (see below) and are considered to be a medical condition with potential life-threatening complications.

SLEEP APNOEA

Derived from the Greek, 'apnoea' means 'want of breath' and refers to a temporary inability to breathe during sleep. The actual causes of sleep apnoea are uncertain, but the problem is primarily associated with obesity, as well as high blood pressure, coronary heart disease, strokes and other cardiovascular problems, and constitutes one of the largest areas of research into sleep disorders.

The onset of sleep is usually accompanied by mild to severe snoring, with short interruptions of breathing at any point during the five phases of sleep. At the point at which the snoring ceases, so too does the breathing. Anything longer than a ten-second cessation of breathing is clinically determined to be a case of sleep apnoea, as it is potentially damaging to the brain. The 'apnoeic events' can occur up to 20 or 30 times per night and this condition may require monitoring in hospital.

Understandably, fatigued sufferers often tend to fall asleep during the day and experience frequent headaches. Alcohol consumption and smoking have both been found to exacerbate the severity and frequency of sleep apnoea.

Treatment for sleep apnoea is complex, involving physical therapies and in some cases surgery to open up restricted air passages. It is unlikely that diet and nutrition alone would be at the root of the problem, but it is always worth considering food intolerances (see p.96).

NARCOLEPSY

Narcolepsy is a chronic, rare sleep disorder with no known cause, characterized by sudden and uncontrollable episodes of deep sleep. Symptoms include overwhelming drowsiness during the day, and apparent chronic fatigue, with sufferers falling asleep on the phone or even at the driving wheel. Sexual problems, such as loss of libido (see pp.54 and 59) and impotence (see p.52), are sometimes additional complications of fatigue.

In many cases of snoring, dairy foods were the sole contributory factor.

More serious symptoms include 'cataplexy', or sudden paralysing episodes of loss of muscle function, limp limbs or an inability to speak clearly. These attacks can be triggered by sudden emotional reactions, such as anger, laughter or fear. A cataplexic attack may last from several seconds to several minutes, but in all cases the person remains conscious.

Hypnagogic phases of sleep (these occur during the first stage of sleep, see p.67) may also occur, in which vivid, often frightening, dream-like experiences happen during the dozing or falling-asleep stage. Sleep paralysis is another symptom of narcolepsy, where the person suffers from a temporary inability to talk or move when falling asleep or waking up. All of these more serious symptoms may occur in people who are not actually suffering from narcolepsy, but if they happen more than once or twice, medical advice should be sought. Interestingly, it is the length of non-REM and REM sleep patterns that are disturbed in narcolepsy. The normal length of non-REM phases of sleep is approximately 90 minutes, followed by the REM or dreaming stage. In narcolepsy this pattern is reversed, with the REM phase at the beginning and immobility or alterations in muscle weakness from the normal patterns.

Treatment includes the encouragement of short periods of napping, with some drug administration in severe cases. Active family involvement is essential, and as a result it can be disruptive to normal family life. Thankfully, it is a relatively rare sleep disorder, compared to sleep apnoea.

FATIGUE SYNDROMES

These two fatigue syndromes, with widely differing causes, are becoming increasingly common.

TATT (TIRED ALL THE TIME SYNDROME)

This widespread syndrome usually occurs as a result of poor eating habits, when stimulants such as tea, coffee and alcohol are consumed regularly throughout the day and highly sugared snacks form a large part of the diet. Symptoms include: frequent yawning, general lethargy, physical fatigue, dark circles under the eyes, irritability, mood swings, emotional outbursts, loss of sex drive and lack of concentration.

CHRONIC FATIGUE SYNDROME (ALSO KNOWN AS M.E. OR MYALGIC ENCEPHALOMYELITIS)

This chronic condition usually results from a viral attack that leaves the person completely debilitated and unable to recover their energy (hence its alternative name of Post-Viral Fatigue Syndrome). It can affect a person's energy levels so intensely that they may be confined to bed for weeks or even months on end. Dietary implications are rarely involved, although some people have found that completely eliminating wheat products effects considerable change. This may be due to the high gluten content of wheat, which may inhibit the absorption of vital nutrients. Symptoms of Chronic Fatigue Syndrome include: complete exhaustion, falling asleep regularly (sometimes even during an activity), loss of appetite, depression, total physical weakness, loss of concentration and memory, lack of motivation and crying for no apparent reason.

SLEEP SUPPLEMENTS

We should be able to get all the nutrients we require for sound sleep from the foods that we eat in our daily diet. As you become more aware of which foods contain which nutrients, you can boost your intake of those that may be useful to enhance sleep. Very occasionally, however, you may need to take either nutritional supplements or herbal remedies.

B VITAMINS

B vitamins (see p.77) comprise perhaps the most important group of nutrients required to combat insomnia. Although they are generally found in common foods, there may be increased requirements for many reasons, which if not met will result in deficiencies. Supplementing vitamin B6 can have significant results in preventing insomnia, while vitamin B3 is believed to be have qualities usually found in the benzodiazepine family of sleeping pills – a fact that highlights its potential in promoting sleep. Vitamin B1 is also required to help avoid insomnia. Supplementation of B vitamins is not recommended for everyone, however, and it is not advisable to take individual B vitamins in isolation; instead, choose a B-complex supplement that contains the full range of this essential group of nutrients.

MAGNESIUM AND CALCIUM

These minerals work synergistically with one another. Calcium is responsible for the contraction of muscles, whilst magnesium relaxes them. Deficiencies in either of these minerals can result in tension, muscle cramps or an inability to relax. Both magnesium and calcium are found in fish, nuts and seeds and especially dark green vegetables (magnesium being a significant component of chlorophyll, the vivid green substance found in plants). Ensuring that your diet is rich in these foods will increase your chances of getting an undisturbed night's sleep.

CHROMIUM

If you often wake in the night feeling alert and unable to get back to sleep, taking 200mcg of chromium (either in picolinate or polynicotinate form) last thing at night can help to balance your blood-sugar levels throughout the night. If you are already taking supplements that contain chromium in any form, then do not exceed 600mcg from all sources in any 24-hour period.

MELATONIN

As we have seen (p.95), melatonin is thought to increase the quality of sleep, and there is some anecdotal evidence to suggest that is particularly effective in older people. It is considered safe to use on occasions, and in small doses (usually 1–3mg at night). Side-effects may include day-after drowsiness, headaches and itching. Melatonin is not available in the UK as no products have a license. However, it is freely available in the United States in health stores and pharmacies.

TRYPTOPHAN

This amino acid is responsible for promoting sleep, as it is converted into serotonin (see p.95). It is found naturally in bananas, figs, cottage cheese, eggs, milk, dried dates, halibut, seaweed, beef and turkey. Perhaps there is some basis for suggesting warm milk at bedtime after all, although if its efficacy is indeed due to its tryptophan content, then it follows that a banana or a slice of turkey should have the same effect. Tryptophan is also available in supplement form, and was easy to buy for many years. In the UK, the **British National Formulary** restricts tryptophan to use by hospital specialists only, and close and regular surveillance is required. Tryptophan is still available in some countries in northern Europe, although supplementing it is not advisable without medical or nutritional supervision. It can have some lingering after-effects, such as continued dizziness and lethargy, and should be treated with caution.

There is an alternative that has gained popularity in recent years. The human body converts tryptophan into a substance known as 5-hydroxytryptophan (5-HTP), the immediate precursor to serotonin, and it is possible to supplement this derivative directly – 5-hydroxytrptophan is reputed to be effective at calming the CNS and promoting sleep, although it has yet to be fully researched. Anecdotal evidence suggests that it is safe, but as with all sleep aids, dosages should be low at first, and users should be vigilant in noting after-affects such as drowsiness the next day or continued fatigue after use. Do not take tryptophan without consulting a doctor as it can interact with some types of anti-depressants.

HERBAL REMEDIES

Herbal sleep remedies have long been popular and are considered a 'safe' alternative to medication. In most cases they can be highly effective, but – like medicinal sleeping pills – they can have side-effects and should ideally be used to promote sleep on an occasional basis. It is preferable to identify and address the underlying causes of insomnia and not simply to rely on pills – herbal or otherwise.

Valerian (**Valeriana officinalis**) also known as 'all-heal', is one of the best-selling herbs in the United States. It contains valepotriates and valerianic acid, although the active ingredient of the herb has still not been identified. It calms the CNS and causes muscle relaxation, and although it is considered to be safe, there is a question mark over the varying qualities of the most popular brands. If you choose to use sleeping remedies containing valerian, consider starting with doses lower than those suggested on the packet, and build up the dose as required without exceeding the manufacturer's recommended levels.

Ginseng (various species of **Panax**) can be found in a number of varieties, including American, Asian, Vietnamese and Korean. Each has subtle differences, yet most have some effect in inducing sleep. Ginseng can actually stimulate and relax the CNS and is known as an adaptogen. It should ideally be taken for three months maximum and then have a break, but should not be used if you have hypertension. Some regular users experience a mild nervousness and anxiety on first taking the herb, although this generally passes as tolerance increases. If you experience any side-effects, we suggest that you lower the dose and build up again slowly.

Kava kava is cultivated from a shrub (**Piper methysticum**) that grows in Polynesia. It has many therapeutic qualities, not least that it is believed to calm anxiety, stress and restlessness – all underlying influences in insomnia. Kava kava contains compounds known as kava lactones, and is believed to induce sleep and relax the muscles. There have been several research projects that have provided positive evidence that this herb is effective in treating insomnia, although studies have suggested that it should not be used in conjunction with any other agents that affect the CNS.

Hops (**Humulus lupulus**) contain a number of substances that have a mild sedative-like effect on the CNS. They contain valerianic acid, which induces relaxation, thus promoting sleep. Hops are considered most effective when taken 45 minutes before retiring, and perhaps best taken as a tincture added to water. The usual adult dose is 2.5–5ml. Hops are generally not suggested if you suffer from clinical depression.

recipe

Foods to help you eat your way to

better sex and sle

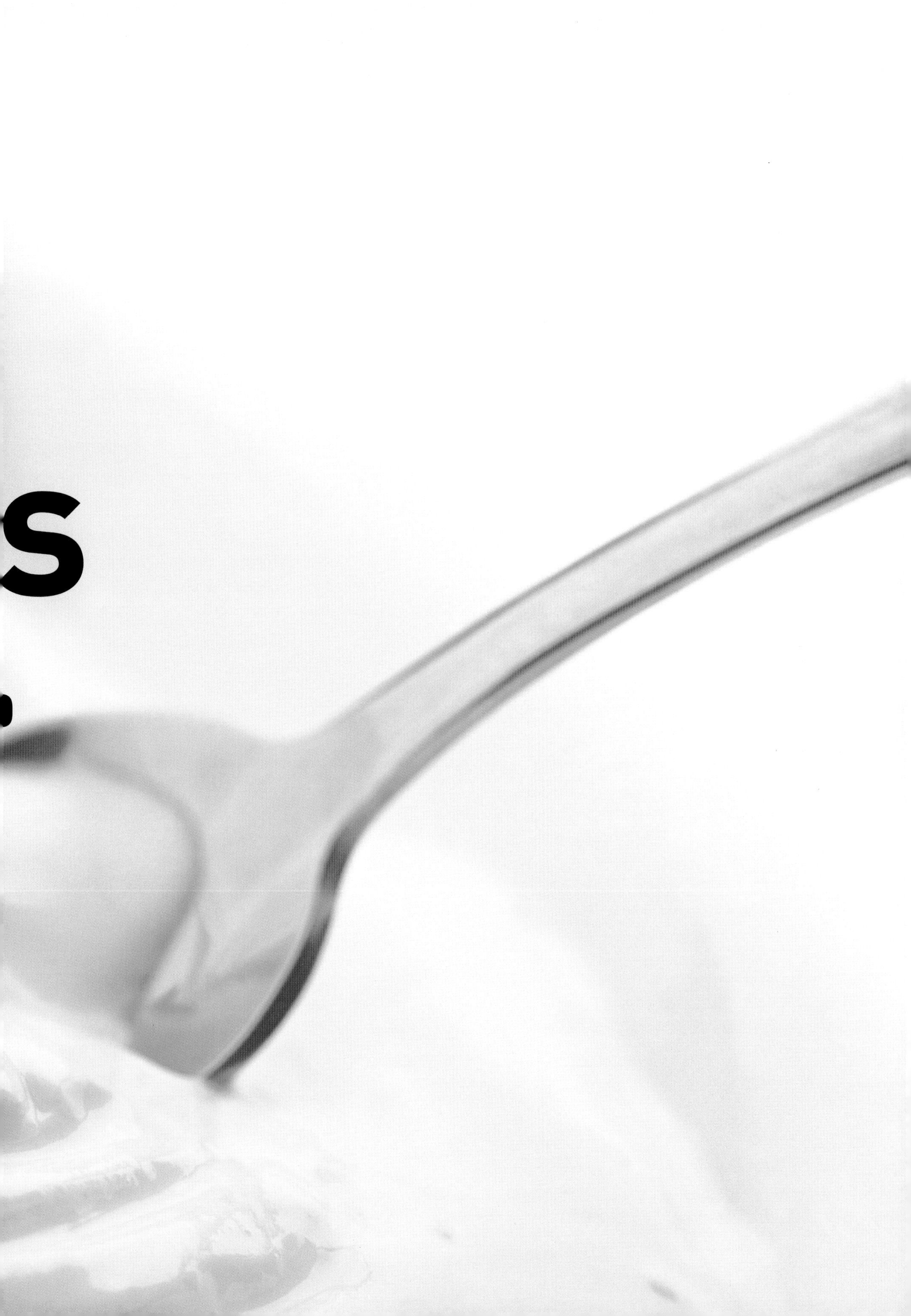

sexy recipes

The primary requirements for an active and healthy sex life are undoubtedly plenty of energy and stamina. The foods included in the following recipes have been selected for their ability to balance blood-sugar levels and produce maximum energy as well as providing the necessary nutrients for optimal sexual function. All recipes serve two unless otherwise stated.

Raspberry and Mango Smoothie

Smoothies are an excellent combination of protein and carbohydrates – essential for keeping hormonal levels balanced. Of all the berries, raspberries contain just about the most nutrients, are very digestible and particularly beneficial for female hormonal conditions. Mangoes are rich in vitamin C, which helps the body to cope with stress. Drink the smoothie within half an hour of making it, as exposure to air rapidly diminishes its nutrient value.

2oz/50g/⅓C pumpkin seeds
7oz/200g/1½C organic plain tofu, drained and cubed
3½oz/100g/⅓C raspberries, fresh or frozen
1 mango, peeled and de-stoned
25 fl oz/750ml/3C rice milk, oat milk or soya milk
1 tbsp/1½ tbsp plain live organic yoghurt (optional)

Place the pumpkin seeds in a blender or food processor and grind for 30 seconds. Add the remaining ingredients. Blend until smooth and serve immediately.

Creamy Porridge with Prunes

Oats are a wonderfully comforting food and are known for their calming effect on the nerves – essential in helping to combat stress. Oats and prunes both provide energy, as well as help to regulate hormones. Add some ground pumpkin and sesame seeds when cooked for even more energy.

43oz/85g/1C organic rolled oats
30fl oz/850ml/3¾C water
5 prunes, soaked overnight in enough water to cover them
2 tbsp/⅓C yoghurt
1 level tbsp pumpkin or sesame seeds, ground (1 heaped tbsp ready ground)

Soak the oats in the water, overnight if possible, for extra creaminess and digestibility. Chop the prunes into small pieces and add them with their soaking water to a saucepan, together with the oats and their water. Bring to the boil, stirring continuously. Simmer for 10 minutes, stirring them to prevent sticking and adding more water if the porridge becomes too thick. Remove from the heat and allow to stand for a few minutes. Add a generous dollop of yoghurt and a sprinkling of the seeds and serve at once.

Baked Eggs with Spinach

Eggs are a great source of protein for starting the day and keeping your energy levels up. They contain choline, one of the B vitamins responsible for providing energy and the feel-good factor. Spinach is high in various nutrients, being packed full of iron for energy and B vitamins for combating stress. Altogether this makes a perfect way to start the day.

1 tbsp/1½ tbsp extra-virgin olive oil
8oz/225g fresh spinach, washed
½ level tsp sea salt
sprinkling of grated nutmeg
2 free-range eggs
black pepper

Preheat the oven to 400°F/205°C/gas mark 6. Heat the oil in a large pan, then add the spinach and salt. Cover and cook on a low heat for 5 minutes. Remove the lid and cook until almost no liquid remains. Drain the spinach, chop it finely and allow to cool.

Lightly grease 2 ramekin dishes with buttered paper and sprinkle each one with nutmeg. Divide the spinach between the ramekins. Make a well in the spinach and crack an egg into each well. Bake for 10–15 minutes, grind over some black pepper and serve immediately.

Bean-Sprout and Pumpkin-Seed Salad

Bean-sprouts are packed with nutrients, particularly vitamins B and C, iron and potassium, all of which are important for sustaining energy and combating stress. Pumpkin seeds are packed with zinc, which is vital for sperm formation and motility, thereby increasing fertility.

1oz/25g/¼C pumpkin seeds
pinch of sea salt
8oz/250g/2½C mixed bean-sprouts, such as mung, alfalfa, lentil and chickpea (if available)
2 whole spring onions (scallions), finely chopped
½ avocado, peeled and cut into cubes
1 sheet nori seaweed (or crisp lettuce leaves)
1 level tbsp nori flakes (or fresh parsley, finely chopped)
large handful of fresh coriander (cilantro)

For the dressing;
3oz/85g/½C tofu
2 tbsp/2½ tbsp extra-virgin olive oil
3fl oz/75ml/¼C water
1 tbsp/1½ tbsp tamari or rich soy sauce
1 small red chilli, seeded and finely chopped (optional)
1 clove garlic, crushed
juice of ½ lime
salt and freshly ground black pepper

Dry-roast the pumpkin seeds in a small frying pan over a high flame, with some sea salt but no additional oil. Mix together the bean-sprouts, spring onions (scallions) and avocado and set aside.

Blend all the dressing ingredients together until absolutely smooth. Add half of the dressing to the salad and mix well. Place a sheet of seaweed (or a couple of lettuce leaves) on a plate, pile the salad on top in a mound and garnish with the rest of the dressing, the nori flakes (or parsley) and the coriander (cilantro).

Watercress, Orange and Sesame-Seed Salad

Watercress is high in vitamin C – the prime nutrient for coping with stress – as are oranges. The high iron and iodine content of watercress also makes it very helpful for hormonal problems, especially for improving thyroid function, regulating energy and increasing sex drive.

1 large bunch watercress, washed very thoroughly
1 orange, peeled and segmented
3 tbsp/¼C extra-virgin olive oil
2 tbsp/2½ tbsp lemon juice
salt and pepper
1oz/25g/¼C toasted sesame seeds (or substitute pumpkin seeds, if desired, but increase the quantity to 4oz/115g/1C)

Chop the stalks of the watercress into 1in/2.5cm pieces and place them with the watercress leaves in a bowl, together with the orange segments. Combine the olive oil, lemon juice and seasoning, then pour this dressing over the salad. Mix well, then sprinkle over the sesame or pumpkin seeds.

Salade Niçoise

Both tuna and anchovies are a good source of omega-3 essential fatty acids, selenium and zinc – all excellent nutrients for providing energy, boosting libido and protecting you against a stressful lifestyle. Tuna is also high in tryptophan, a natural mood improver. The combination of tuna and eggs provides first-class protein, eggs also being high in choline, which is important for balancing the hormones and improving mood. With its nutrient-rich salad combinations providing extra energy, this recipe makes a perfectly balanced lunchtime salad or light supper.

1 head of cos lettuce (or similar), washed and dried
2 small free-range eggs, hardboiled and quartered
1 beef tomato, washed and quartered
½ large red pepper, seeded and quartered
½ cucumber, peeled and sliced
2 medium-sized waxy potatoes, boiled, refreshed in cold water and diced
12 black olives, halved and stoned
3½ oz/100g can of tuna, in brine, drained and flaked
4 anchovy fillets

For the dressing:
3 tbsp/¼C extra-virgin olive oil
1½ tbsp/2 tbsp good wine vinegar or balsamic vinegar
3 rounded tsp finely chopped mixed fresh herbs, such as basil and parsley
1 clove garlic, finely chopped

Line the salad bowl with the lettuce leaves. Pile all the other ingredients in the middle and arrange the anchovy fillets on top. Mix gently together with your fingers.

To make the dressing, combine the olive oil, vinegar, herbs and garlic. Pour over the salad just before eating.

Fennel, Apple and Almond Salad

Fennel is rich in phyto-oestrogens, which are very helpful in treating female hormonal complaints – primarily the menopause. Almonds are a fantastic source of magnesium, which is important for nerve transmission in order to increase sexual enjoyment, and of essential fatty acids for the production of sex hormones. And apples contain vitamin C, for stress management.

- 3 tbsp/½C live yoghurt
- 3 tbsp/½C light mayonnaise
- 2 tbsp/2½ tbsp lemon juice
- salt and pepper
- 1 small apple, peeled, cored and diced
- 1 small fennel bulb, trimmed and diced
- handful of almonds, finely chopped
- handful of fresh herbs, such as parsley or coriander (cilantro), finely chopped

Stir together the yoghurt, light mayonnaise and lemon juice, then season to taste with salt and pepper. Mix the apple and fennel together with the dressing. Check the seasoning. Scatter some almonds over the top and the herbs of your choice.

Brown Rice and Pumpkin-Seed Salad

Brown rice is abundant in B vitamins and zinc, both of which are essential for maintaining energy levels and sustaining sex drive. Pumpkin seeds are one of the most nourishing foods for the male prostate gland and are vital for helping to balance the hormones.

- 4oz/125g/½C short-grain brown rice
- 16 fl oz/500ml/2C water
- 2 tbsp/2½ tbsp olive oil
- handful of fresh mint leaves, finely chopped
- handful of fresh flat-leaf parsley leaves, finely chopped
- 3 level tbsp/¼C spring onions (scallions), finely sliced
- half a cucumber. peeled, seeded and diced
- 3 tbsp/¼C lemon juice
- black pepper
- 2oz/50g/½C pumpkin seeds
- 250g/8½oz halloumi cheese

Rinse the rice thoroughly in plenty of cold running water. Put it in a saucepan with the water and bring to the boil, covered. Turn down the heat to a simmer and cook until all the water has been absorbed (about 40 minutes). Turn off the heat and leave the rice to stand.

Put all the remaining ingredients apart from the halloumi into a bowl and mix thoroughly. When the rice has cooled a little, but is still just warm, add it to the bowl and mix well.

Heat the grill until hot. Slice the cheese lengthways to a thickness of about ½in/1cm and grill the slices until they are a rich brown on each side. Serve with the rice salad.

Miso Soup

Miso is a fermented food made from soya beans and grains, to which an enzymatic culture has been added. It is a superb source of easily assimilated protein, and is rich in nutrients. Miso contains a high proportion of B vitamins to aid the nervous system, act as a stress-buster and provide the energy that is essential for sex. It can be obtained in health-food and Japanese stores.

16 fl oz/500ml/2C water
2oz/60g/½C miso
1 tbsp/1½ tbsp tamari or rich soy sauce
toasted sesame seeds, to garnish
spring onions (scallions), sliced paper-thin, to garnish

Options:
sautéed mushrooms, grated carrot, tofu

Heat the water in a pan to just below simmering point. In a bowl dissolve the miso with one-quarter of the hot water. Stir this into the pan and mix well. It is very important that the soup never boils once the miso has been added. Flavour to taste with the tamari. Garnish with the sesame seeds and spring onions (scallions), and serve at once.

If you want a more varied soup, add some sautéed mushrooms and thinly grated carrots at the last minute. Or cut some tofu into bite-sized cubes and simmer it in the broth before serving.

Grapefruit and Vegetable Gazpacho

Grapefruit contains a potent flavonoid called naringin, which has been shown to cleanse the blood as well as being excellent for the cardiovascular system by lowering cholesterol and protecting the arteries from plaque. It thereby increases energy, staying power and, ultimately, sexual performance. This unusual cold soup is very light, refreshing and easily digested.

2 grapefruit, peeled, pips removed and quartered
2 tomatoes, halved and seeded
1 cucumber, peeled, seeded and cut into chunks
2 celery stalks (leaves included)
1 red or green pepper, cut into chunks
handful of fresh parsley
1 small green chilli, seeded (optional)
salt
grapefruit juice, as needed

Purée the grapefruit quarters in a food processor or blender, then pour into a large bowl. Purée the tomatoes and cucumbers and add to the grapefruit purée. Purée the remaining solid ingredients and add to the bowl, with salt and grapefruit juice as needed. Stir well and chill the soup in the refrigerator before serving.

Cabbage Parcels with Red Lentils and Sweet Onions

Lentils and cabbage are good sources of choline, one of the B vitamins essential for energy and therefore, indirectly, for boosting libido. Lentils are also packed with zinc and manganese, both of which are useful for increasing sexual performance. Cabbage also stimulates the liver and is high in indoles, which are helpful in balancing the female hormones.

3½oz/100g/½C red lentils
salt
1 small Savoy cabbage
2 medium-sized onions, halved and sliced
3 tbsp/¼C extra-virgin olive oil
2 tbsp/2½ tbsp honey
grated zest and juice of 1 large lemon
freshly ground black pepper

Wash the lentils, place them in a small lidded saucepan and cover with cold water. Bring to the boil and skim off the foam. Let them boil rapidly for 10 minutes, stirring them from time to time, then reduce the heat to a simmer, add a pinch of salt and cover. You may need to add a little more water if they seem to be drying out. Simmer for about 15 minutes, stirring and checking that they are not burning on the bottom. The resulting consistency should look like porridge.

Meanwhile put a large pot of salted water on to boil. Cut the cabbage leaves carefully away from the core, discarding the outermost leaves if they look tough. Shave off any thick stems. Blanch the leaves in boiling water for 2 minutes, then refresh them in cold water and leave to drain.

Sauté the onions with a third of the olive oil until they start to brown. Add the honey and stir until nicely caramelized. Combine the onions, cooked lentils, lemon juice and zest. Taste and correct the seasoning.

Preheat the oven to 350°F/180°C/gas mark 4 and oil a baking dish. Pat dry a cabbage leaf. Place a heaped tablespoon of lentil mixture in the middle, near the base of the leaf. Fold over the sides, then roll the leaf up. Place seam-side down in the baking dish to keep the parcel intact. Brush lightly with some of the remaining olive oil. Repeat until all the leaves and mixture have been used up. Bake for 20–25 minutes until lightly browned. Serve hot, warm or cold.

Ginger and Pineapple Chicken

Chicken is an excellent form of low-fat protein and contains the full gamut of B vitamins that are essential for energy production and stress management. Ginger is renowned for its aphrodisiac qualities and, as a stimulant, promotes circulation, thereby boosting energy levels when you feel fatigued or lethargic. Pineapple juice contains vitamin C, for further control of stress.

For the marinade:

5 fl oz/150ml/⅔C unsweetened pineapple juice
⅓ glass dry white wine
1 heaped tbsp finely chopped fresh root ginger
2 tbsp/2½ tbsp wholegrain mustard
1 tbsp/1½ tbsp soy sauce
1 tsp toasted sesame oil or extra-virgin olive oil
1 spring onion (scallion), chopped
1 clove garlic, finely chopped

2 whole boneless, skinless chicken breasts, cut in half

To make the marinade, blend until creamy. Reserve half the marinade for the sauce.

Arrange the chicken pieces in a dish large enough to hold them in a single layer. Pour over the marinade, cover and refrigerate for 2–3 hours or overnight.

Preheat the grill to low.

Remove the chicken from the marinade, keeping this for basting. Place the chicken on the grill rack and cook, basting once or twice, for 6–8 minutes or until the meat is tender and brown.

To make the sauce, bring the reserved marinade to the boil and cook over a high heat for about 10 minutes until it thickens slightly.

Spoon the sauce over the chicken and serve with a mixture of vegetables, such as steamed broccoli, pak choi and spring cabbage.

Grilled Tuna with Mint and Parsley Salsa

A great source of important essential fatty acids, as well as being packed with the potent antioxidants selenium and zinc, and the energy sources in its B vitamins and co-enzyme Q10, tuna is a great protein to include regularly in the diet, especially for improving stamina and libido. Chillies, in moderation, have a mild stimulatory effect, and while improving the circulation may also heighten sensitivity and arousal. They also contain huge amounts of vitamin C, which is vital for stress management.

For the salsa:
small handful of fresh mint leaves
small handful of fresh parsley
1 red chilli, seeded
2 tbsp/2½ tbsp extra-virgin olive oil
2 tbsp/2½ tbsp lemon juice
1 tsp warm water

For the tuna:
2 very fresh tuna steaks, cut 1in/2.5cm thick
extra-virgin olive oil for brushing the fish
freshly ground black pepper

Put all the salsa ingredients into a food processor and blend, but keep the mixture quite chunky.

Place a ridged griddle pan over a high heat or turn on the grill to get really hot.
Brush one side of the tuna with olive oil and grind over plenty of black pepper. Place the oiled side down on the grill pan or face-up under the grill and cook until the fish begins to go opaque at the edges (about 2–3 minutes). Brush the other side of the fish with oil and season with black pepper as before. Cook for a further 1–2 minutes. Serve with a generous helping of the salsa and with freshly steamed vegetables of your choice, such as broccoli, courgettes (zucchini) or French beans.

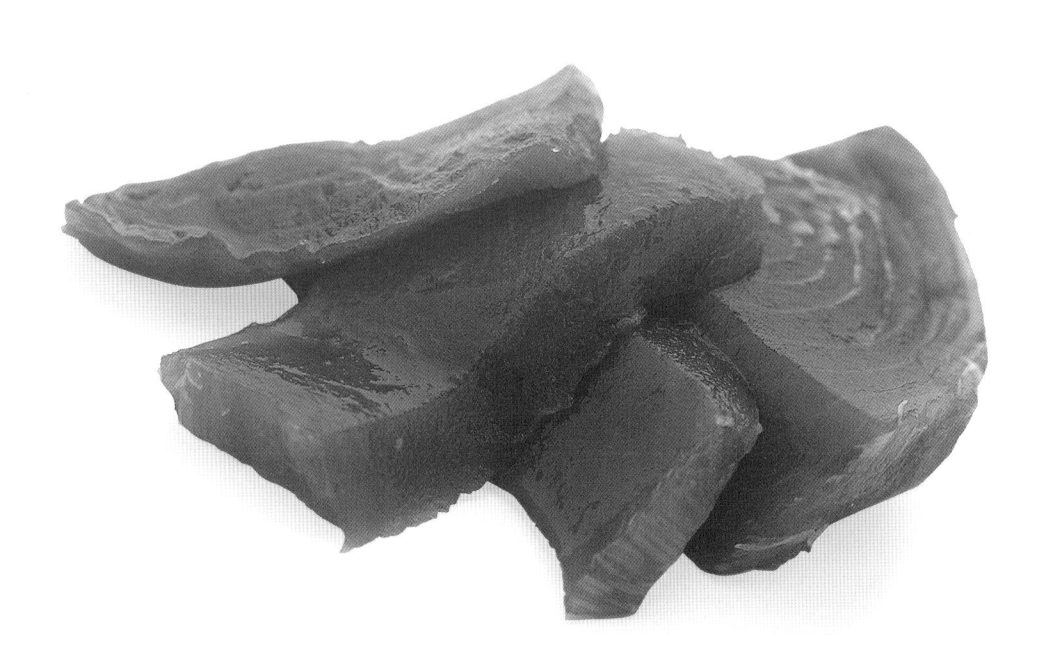

Warm Shellfish Salad with Pine Nuts and Asparagus

All shellfish, especially prawns (shrimp), contain enormous amounts of zinc, which is essential for a high sperm count and increased libido. Asparagus has long been considered an aphrodisiac, possibly in part due to its shape! Because of its incredibly supportive action on the liver, it can help regulate hormonal balance and therefore aids sexual function. Pine nuts contain B vitamins and magnesium for sustaining energy and vitality.

4 large fresh asparagus spears
11/2oz/45g mangetout, topped and tailed
large handful of rocket (arugula) and/or mixed salad greens, thoroughly washed
2 tbsp/2½ tbsp chopped fresh coriander (cilantro)
½ level tsp five-spice powder
½ fresh red chilli, seeded and finely chopped (optional)
1 clove garlic, crushed
4 medium-sized fresh prawns (shrimp), peeled and de-veined
4 scallops
3 tbsp/¼ C extra-virgin olive oil
2 spring onions (scallions), sliced
2 tsp lemon juice
1 tbsp/1½ tbsp tamari or rich soy sauce
1 tbsp/1½ tbsp sesame oil
1 level tbsp pine nuts, lightly toasted
1 level tsp sesame seeds

Steam the asparagus until tender (about 4 minutes, depending on its thickness) and then refresh in cold water. Blanch the mangetout in boiling water for 30 seconds, then drain and refresh in cold water. Arrange the rocket (arugula), asparagus and mangetout on a plate.

Mix together three-quarters of the coriander (cilantro), the five-spice powder, chilli (if desired) and garlic. Add the prawns (shrimp) and scallops to the spice mix and toss lightly. Heat most of the olive oil in a wok or heavy-based saucepan and, when it is hot, add the seafood and spring onions (scallions) and cook over a high heat for 1–3 minutes until opaque. Be careful not to overcook them or the scallops will become rubbery. Remove and place the seafood on top of the salad greens.

Add the remaining olive oil, lemon juice and tamari to the wok until sizzling. At the last minute add sesame oil to taste. Drizzle the dressing over the salad, sprinkle with pine nuts, sesame seeds and the remaining coriander (cilantro) and serve while still warm.

Salmon with Sultanas, Ginger and Pine Nuts

Salmon is a good source of omega-3 essential fatty acids, which are important for balancing the hormones and heightening sexual arousal. In addition, pine nuts are rich in zinc for healthy sperm production and staying power, and ginger has long been hailed for having aphrodisiac qualities.

1 level tbsp sultanas
juice of 1 lemon
2 x 41/2oz/125g salmon fillets
black pepper
2 level tbsp pine nuts
handful of fresh coriander (cilantro)
1 level tbsp thinly sliced fresh ginger

Put the sultanas in a small bowl and pour over enough boiling water to cover them. Leave to soak until plump (about 15 minutes).

Preheat the oven to its hottest setting. Oil a baking tray and place it in the oven. Squeeze the lemon juice over all sides of the fish and grind over black pepper to taste.

Put the drained sultanas, pine nuts, coriander (cilantro) and ginger in a small bowl and, using kitchen scissors, roughly cut them up. Divide the mixture in two, arranging it on top of each salmon fillet. Place on the hot baking tray and bake in the oven for about 15 minutes or until the fish is opaque (depending on its thickness). Serve with a cooling herbed green salad and brown rice.

Spinach-Stuffed Mushrooms

Both mushrooms and spinach are packed with energy-providing nutrients – mushrooms, in particular, with B vitamins and zinc, both of which are essential for increased vitality and staying power.

5oz/140g/1¼C fresh spinach, washed thoroughly
grating of nutmeg
salt and pepper
4 large, flat mushrooms, cleaned
2 tbsp/2½ tbsp extra-virgin olive oil
2 cloves garlic, finely sliced
1oz/30g/⅓C dried breadcrumbs
1oz/30g/⅓C Parmesan cheese, freshly grated

Preheat the oven to 400°F/205°C/gas mark 6. Lightly shake the spinach to remove some of the water, then place it in a pan (with no added water) over a high heat until wilted and tender (about 2 minutes). Remove from the pan and, in a colander, squeeze out all the excess water. Chop finely and mix with a generous grating of nutmeg and salt and pepper to taste.

Place the mushrooms side by side, top down, in a shallow baking tray. Divide the spinach mixture into 4 and place a portion on top of each mushroom. Mix half the olive oil with the garlic, breadcrumbs and Parmesan and place on top of the spinach mixture. Drizzle the remaining oil over and around the mushrooms. Place them in the oven for 15 minutes, until they are sizzling and the breadcrumb mixture is well browned. Serve with quinoa and steamed green beans.

Broad Bean (Fava Bean), Pea and Asparagus Risotto

Broad beans (fava beans) and peas are an excellent source of vegetarian protein and fibre – peas in particular being helpful in controlling blood-sugar levels, and thus in increasing energy and vitality. Asparagus is known to be very supportive of the liver, which has a role in regulating the sex hormones.

25 fl oz/750ml/3C vegetable stock
2 tbsp/2½ tbsp extra-virgin olive oil
1 medium-sized onion, finely chopped
5oz/140g/1C peas, fresh or frozen
5oz/140g/1½C broad beans (fava beans), fresh or frozen
2 cloves garlic, finely chopped
6oz/170g/1C Arborio rice
1 glass dry white wine (optional)
3oz/90g asparagus, chopped
3 tbsp/¼C flat-leaf (Italian) parsley
handful of grated Parmesan cheese (optional)
salt and freshly ground pepper

Bring the stock to the boil and keep it simmering gently. Heat the olive oil in a heavy saucepan and sauté the onion until pale gold and soft. If using fresh peas and beans, add them to the saucepan at this stage with the garlic (if using frozen peas and beans, blanch them in salted water for 2 minutes, then refresh them in cold water and add them a few minutes before the rice is done).

Cook the vegetables over a low heat for 2 minutes, stir well then add the rice and the wine (if desired) and stir for 1–2 minutes to coat the rice. Add the hot stock, a ladleful at a time, stirring continuously until it has all been absorbed. Repeat until the rice is al dente and creamy in texture. Meanwhile, blanch the asparagus in salted water for 1 minute.

Just before serving the rice, add the parsley, Parmesan and asparagus, and check the seasoning. Leave to stand, covered, for 5 minutes. Serve with a large green salad.

Honey-Drizzled Figs with Vanilla Yoghurt

Figs have always been recognized as a sexy fruit – rightly so, with their high levels of beta-carotene and vitamin C, which are useful for increasing energy, sex-hormone production and consequently libido. They are also excellent for supporting blood-sugar management.

6 ripe figs, soft to the touch and oozing nectar
3 tsp runny honey
6 tbsp vanilla or plain yoghurt

Gently but thoroughly wash the figs. Peel back the skin from the tip to halfway down. Evenly drizzle some honey over each fig and spoon yoghurt generously over the top.

Banana Custard

Bananas are high in potassium, which benefits the muscular and nervous system, leading to elevated mood, increased stamina and well-being and in turn increased libido and sex drive. The eggs in the custard are high in choline, one of the B vitamins that enhance mood and energy.

yolks of 2 medium free-range eggs
½ tsp cornflour (cornstarch)
10 fl oz/300ml/1¼C goat's milk, sheep's milk, soya milk or rice milk
1 tsp vanilla extract or a vanilla pod
1 tbsp honey
2 ripe bananas

Put the egg yolks and cornflour (cornstarch) into a bowl large enough to hold the milk as well. Set aside.

In a heavy-based saucepan, heat the milk with the vanilla extract or pod to boiling point. Remove from the heat, extract the vanilla pod (if used) and whisk in the honey with a balloon whisk. Cool for 5 minutes.

Break up the egg yolks with the whisk and pour the milk mixture over them, whisking all the time – if the milk is too hot, the eggs will scramble! Return the mixture to the saucepan and, over a low heat and stirring constantly with a wooden spoon, heat until it thickens. Do not allow the custard to boil. As soon as it is the thickness of cream, remove the pan from the heat. Slice the bananas into the custard while it is warm. Pour into individual bowls and when cool chill in the refrigerator.

Exotic Tutti-Frutti Salad

Mango and papaya are both rich in beta-carotene, an important nutrient for the production of sex hormones. And all the fruit in this recipe, particularly the kiwi fruit, contain large amounts of vitamin C, which is the main anti-stress nutrient and of prime importance for increasing sex drive.

1 ripe mango, peeled and cubed
1 ripe papaya, seeded, peeled and cubed
1 kiwi fruit, peeled and sliced into rounds
1 peach, skinned and cubed
8 strawberries, trimmed and cored
large handful of black grapes, halved and seeded
2 tbsp/2½ tbsp fresh double cream (heavy cream)
2 passion fruit
large sprig of fresh mint

Mix all the fruit, except the passion fruit, together, then place a selection in individual bowls. Spoon over a large dollop of fresh cream and squeeze the pips and juice from a passion fruit over each bowl. Decorate with mint and serve.

Rich Chocolate, Walnut and Orange Torte

Chocolate is rich in phenylalanine, a chemical that the brain manufactures which enhances mood and arousal. High in magnesium, chocolate also enhances nerve and muscle transmissions, promoting increased sensitivity and staying power.

14oz/400g/3½C ground walnuts
3½oz/100g/¼C cocoa powder
1 level tsp cardamom seeds, freshly ground
1 level tsp sea salt
2 oranges, washed
8 fl oz/250ml/1C maple syrup
5 medium free-range eggs
whipped cream (optional)

Preheat the oven to 170°C/325°F/gas mark 3. Combine all the dry ingredients in a large bowl.

Wash the oranges and boil whole in water until very soft (about 20 minutes). Remove from the water, drain thoroughly, halve and remove the seeds. Blend the maple syrup and oranges thoroughly in a food processor or blender to create an emulsion or very smooth sauce.

Whisk the eggs to a foamy consistency and blend with the emulsion. Gently fold the wet ingredients into the dry. Pour into a 9in/23cm oiled cake tin. Bake in the oven for approximately 1 hour, or until a knife inserted into the middle comes out clean. Remove from the oven and cool completely before turning out. Serve with whipped cream (if desired).

Green Velvet

Avocado is one of the world's perfect foods. High in beta-carotene (for the production of sex hormones), it also helps balance the hormones with its high phyto-oestrogenic quality, as well as providing essential fats and B vitamins to combat stress and improve libido. Avocados are incredibly versatile and quick to prepare, and may be added to soups and salads or used to make this easy-spreading snack.

2 ripe avocados
1 tbsp/1½ tbsp fresh lemon juice
2 cloves garlic, crushed
2 level tbsp fresh coriander (cilantro), chopped
salt and freshly ground pepper

Cut the avocados in half and remove the stones. Scoop the flesh from the shells into a mixing bowl and mash with a fork. Stir in the remaining ingredients and season to taste. Serve with organic corn chips, rice or oat cakes, or crostini (see below).

Crostini

A delicious garlicky base for serving with dips and assorted garnishes, crostini are quick and easy to prepare. Their garlic content ensures that they have an aphrodisiac element. They may be used as a snack or as a nutritious starter to a main meal.

2 cloves garlic, crushed
2 tbsp/2½ tbsp extra-virgin olive oil
1 good-quality loaf of sourdough rye or sourdough bread

Preheat the oven to 375°F/190°C/gas mark 5. Combine the garlic and olive oil in a bowl and set aside.

Cut the bread into ½in/1cm slices and brush each side with the oil and garlic mixture. Lay the slices flat on an ungreased baking tray, and bake on the centre rack of the oven until the bread begins to crispen, but is still a little chewy (about 10–12 minutes). Remove from the oven and serve hot, warm or at room temperature with the topping of your choice.

Topping suggestions:
Green Velvet (see above)
Goat's cheese with tomato and basil
Mashed hard-boiled egg with grated lemon zest, parsley and ricotta cheese
Cooked prawns (shrimps) with chopped tomatoes, coriander (cilantro) and lemon juice
Hummus topped with alfalfa sprouts
Asparagus spears and Pecorino cheese

Oysters

Oysters must count as the ultimate sexy snack. Containing more zinc than any other seafood, they are rightly known as a serious libido enhancer. They also improve fertility by increasing sperm production. Eat them raw with a squeeze of lemon and a grinding of black pepper – or, if you prefer, add some chopped onion and a dash of Tabasco.

Almond-Stuffed Olives and Dates

Almonds are a rich source of essential fatty acids and magnesium, which are important for the production of sex hormones and for nerve transmission. Dates provide energy due to their high natural sugar content. Olives contain abundant calcium, which is essential for muscle contraction and sensitivity. Medjool dates and Kalamata olives, the fattest, fullest Greek olives, can be found in good supermarkets, health-food stores and delicatessens. The riper the olives, the easier they are to pit and stuff.

2 dozen blanched whole almonds
16 oil-cured or Kalamata olives
8 whole Medjool dates

Preheat the oven to 325°F/160°C/gas mark 3. Spread the almonds on an ungreased baking tray and toast them in the oven until they turn a light golden brown (about 15 minutes). Watch them carefully so that they do not burn. Remove from the oven and leave to cool.

Stone the olives and dates (make a slit at one end of the olive and squeeze – the stone should slip out). Insert one almond into each olive, pushing it in as far as possible and wrapping the olive around it. Repeat the procedure with the remaining almonds and with the dates. Cover tightly and refrigerate until use.

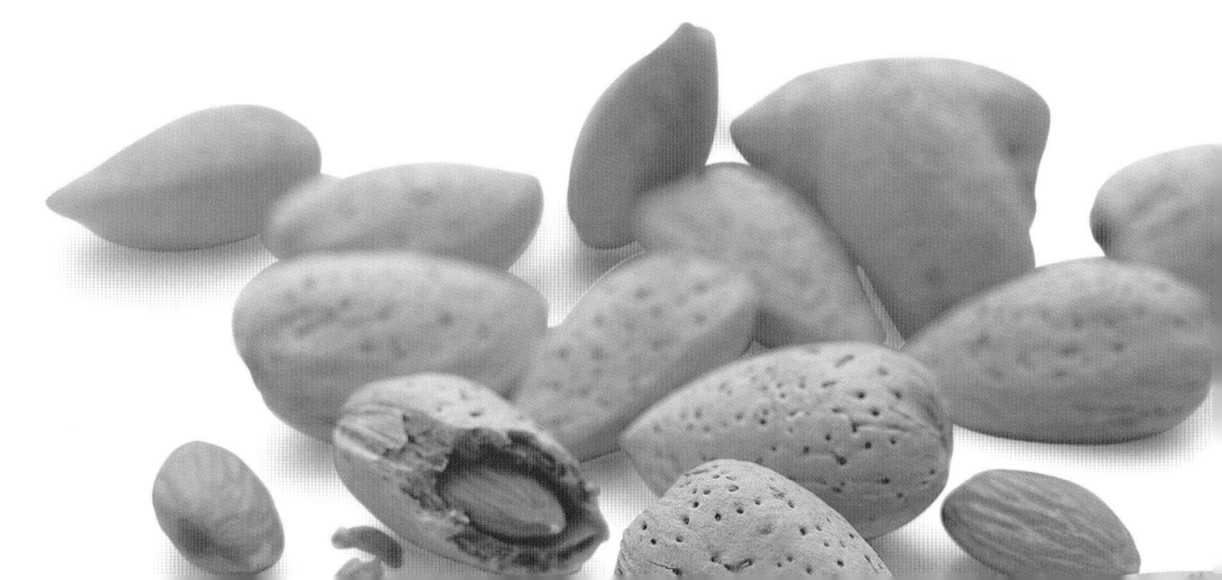

sleepy recipes

It is important to eat consistently throughout the day and then eat lightly in the evenings to avoid overburdening the digestive system and ensure a good night's sleep. Avoid rich or heavy foods that take hours to digest. The following recipes are rich in vitamins and minerals that will encourage proper, restorative sleep. All recipes serve two unless otherwise stated.

Hot Fruit with Ricotta and Cottage Cheese

Stewed fresh or dried fruit makes an excellent way to start the day and provide fibre and vitamin C. With protein from the two cheeses, this dish will provide energy and keep your blood-sugar levels well balanced. If you prefer, substitute yoghurt for the cheeses for a slightly lighter meal.

good handful of dried fruit (apricots, figs, prunes, apples, pears) or fresh fruit (apples, strawberries, apricots, plums)
2 tsp maple syrup or honey (for fresh fruit)

For the topping:
3oz/95g/½C ricotta cheese
3½oz/100g/½C cottage cheese or 8 fl oz/250ml/1C Greek yoghurt

For dried fruit:
Cut the fruit into medium-sized pieces and soak in plenty of water overnight. In a large pan simmer the fruit in their soaking water. Cook over a low heat for 30 minutes, partially covered with a lid. Serve hot.

For fresh fruit:
Do not peel the fruit, but core it and slice into medium or bite-sized pieces. Place in a pan with 4 fl oz/100ml/½C of water (the fruit will produce additional juices) and the honey or maple syrup. Simmer over a low heat for 30 minutes, partially covered with a lid. Serve hot.

To make the topping, mix the ricotta with the cottage cheese and serve in a separate bowl with the stewed fruit. A dollop of the mixture on the hot fruit is delicious. Alternatively, serve some Greek yoghurt.

Feta, Red Pepper and Basil Omelette

Eggs are great for an occasional first-class protein breakfast – say twice a week. They are high in calcium, zinc and B vitamins, all of which are help the body deal with stressful situations.

Makes 2 omelettes
2 tbsp/2½ tbsp extra-virgin olive oil
¼ medium-sized red onion, thinly sliced
salt and pepper
1 clove garlic, finely chopped (optional)
1 medium-sized red pepper, sliced
zest of 1 lemon, grated
2 tsp chopped fresh basil
6 small free-range eggs, beaten
2 tbsp /2½ tbsp water
2oz/50g/⅓C feta cheese, crumbled

Heat about half of the oil in a frying pan. Add the onion, salt and pepper and sauté over a medium heat for 4–5 minutes until the onion is tender. Add the garlic and cook for 1 minute. Add the red pepper and fry gently for a further 3 minutes until it is soft but still has a little bite. Transfer the mixture to a bowl and add the lemon zest and basil.

Season the egg with salt and pepper, then add the water and whisk. Add ½ tsp of the oil to a seasoned omelette pan or small frying pan. When it is sizzling, add half the egg mixture. Using a spatula, move the eggs towards the centre of the pan as they begin to set at the edges. Tilt the pan so that the entire surface is covered with wet eggs. As the eggs begin to set, place half the pepper mixture in the centre, sprinkle with half of the feta, gently fold the omelette over and turn it out onto a plate. Repeat for the second omelette.

Oatmeal Pancakes

Oats are an excellent way to start the day. Not only do they stimulate the digestion and act as a mild laxative, but they are also known for their ability to soothe the nervous system.

Makes approximately 6 4in/10cm pancakes
5 fl oz/150ml/⅔C cow's milk, rice milk or soya milk
2oz/50g/¾C rolled oats
2 tsp extra-virgin olive oil
1 large free-range egg, beaten
1oz/30g/¼C wholewheat flour
1 tsp maple syrup or honey
½ level tsp baking powder
¼ level tsp salt

Combine the milk and oats in a bowl and allow to stand for at least 5 minutes. Add the oil and egg, mixing them well. Stir in the flour, syrup or honey, baking powder and salt. Mix them until the dry ingredients are just moistened.

Using a hot, lightly oiled grill pan or a small pancake pan over a medium heat, pour in one-quarter of the batter for each pancake. Turn the pancake when the top is bubbling and the edges look slightly dry. Serve with a dollop of thick yoghurt and some chopped fresh fruit.

Tuna and Chickpea Salad

Tuna is a great source of protein, benefiting insomniacs by helping to balance blood-sugar levels and providing important B vitamins to support the nervous system and combat stress.

14oz/400g can of chickpeas, salt- and sugar-free
7oz/200g/1⅓C cooked peas, fresh or frozen
7oz/200g/1C tuna, freshly cooked or canned
2 tomatoes, roughly chopped
2 level tbsp each of coarsely chopped fresh basil, chives and parsley
juice of ½ lemon
salt and black pepper
3 tbsp/¼C extra-virgin olive oil
Options: diced avocado, shredded lettuce, sliced radish or cucumber

Rinse the chickpeas under running water and drain them well. Bring a small pan of water to the boil and cook the peas for 5 minutes, then drain them and allow to cool. Slice or flake the tuna.

Mix all the ingredients together in a bowl and serve at room temperature – or chilled, if preferred. For a variation, try adding avocado, lettuce, radish, cucumber or whatever other salad ingredients you have to hand or prefer.

Mangetout, Baby Corn and Asparagus Salad

Due to its fast cooking, this recipe preserves the high quantities of vitamin C, magnesium and calcium present in these vegetables, which can all help contribute to a good night's sleep.

large handful of hiziki seaweed
hot water, to cover seaweed
5 tsp/6 tsp tamari or rich soy sauce
1 heaped tbsp sunflower seeds
1 heaped tbsp sesame seeds
pinch of sea salt
2oz/50g young asparagus, trimmed
1 tbsp/1½ tbsp extra-virgin olive oil
4oz/115g baby corn
3½oz/100g mangetout, topped and tailed
1 tbsp/1½ tbsp water
1–2 tsp umeboshi vinegar (or apple-cider vinegar and a squeeze of fresh lemon juice)
1 x 1in/2.5cm piece of fresh red chilli, finely chopped (optional)
2 level tbsp finely chopped fresh coriander (cilantro) or chives

Soak the seaweed for 15 minutes in hot water with about two-thirds of the tamari, then drain.

Dry-roast the seeds in a pan with some salt over a medium heat until they begin to pop and go golden brown. Set aside.

Bring a small pan of salted water to the boil (a milk pan is large enough), immerse the asparagus and boil for precisely 1 minute. Drain and set aside.

Heat the olive oil in a large frying pan or wok. Add the baby corn and sauté for 3–4 minutes, tossing and turning it all the time until it begins to wilt very slightly and turn golden in places. Add the asparagus and continue to sauté for 30 seconds, then add the mangetout and sauté for a further minute or so. Tossing the ingredients in the pan, quickly add the water (which will sizzle in the heat), the remaining tamari and the umeboshi vinegar (or apple-cider vinegar and lemon juice). Finally add the chilli and the now-tender seaweed. Remove the pan from the heat and add the toasted seeds and some coriander or chives. Serve hot or cold with plain grilled chicken or fish.

Ruby-Red Salad

Beetroot (beet) is renowned for its ability to detoxify the body and cleanse the intestines, aiding digestion – very important for encouraging a good night's sleep. Both beetroot (beet) and cabbage are also high in calcium and magnesium, a good balance of which helps to combat insomnia.

2 small beetroot (beet)
1oz/30g/¼C arame seaweed (kelp or dulse, if arame is unavailable)
8 fl oz/250ml/1C water
3 white cabbage leaves, sliced into bite-sized pieces
1 small red onion, finely sliced
1 bunch radishes, sliced
1 tbsp/1½ tbsp extra-virgin olive oil or cold-pressed, unrefined sesame oil
1 tbsp/1½ tbsp rice vinegar
1 tbsp/1½ tbsp tamari or rich soy sauce
2 level tbsp finely chopped fresh parsley

Slice the beetroot (beet) into thin rounds or grate it, then steam until tender (about 5 minutes). Rinse and soak the arame (or other seaweed) in half the water for 5 minutes, then drain it.

Put the steamed beetroot (beet) into a large mixing bowl with all the other ingredients except the parsley. Stir well and taste. Adjust the seasoning, adding more tamari or soy sauce and/or vinegar, if desired. Sprinkle with the parsley and serve with grilled fish or goat's cheese.

Oriental Pumpkin and Broccoli Salad

Pumpkins and squash are packed with nutrients, including calcium and magnesium, which are needed for sleep. They are some of the mildest and easiest vegetables to digest, making them a perfect light dinner suggestion. They are also valuable in helping to balance blood-sugar levels, due to their rich concentration of slowly metabolized natural sugars. Broccoli, too, contains high levels of important sleep nutrients, while the coconut in this recipe adds a satisfying and comforting creaminess. This dish makes an excellent accompaniment to fish if you add a light green salad.

small handful of hiziki seaweed
3 tbsp/¼C tamari or rich soy sauce
3 cloves garlic, crushed
3 tbsp/¼C extra-virgin olive oil
16oz/450g pumpkin, peeled and cut into 1¼in/3cm chunks
1½in/3cm piece of ginger, peeled and finely minced
5oz/150g broccoli florets, trimmed
4 heaped tbsp roughly chopped fresh coriander (cilantro)
¼ of a fresh coconut, husk removed
1 green chilli, very finely chopped

Place the seaweed in a bowl with a third of the tamari or soy sauce and a half-clove of crushed garlic. Cover with hot water and set aside until soft.

Heat all but 1 tbsp/1½ tbsp of the oil gently, then add the pumpkin. Stir-fry for 3–4 minutes with 2 cloves of the garlic and three-quarters of the minced ginger, turning it over constantly with a wooden spoon until the chunks begin to soften on the outside and mingle with the seasonings. Then add half the remaining tamari or soy sauce, a little at a time, taking care that the pumpkin does not stick or burn. Add a little water if necessary.

Heat the remaining oil in a separate pan and very quickly sauté the broccoli florets with the remaining tamari or soy sauce and the remaining garlic and ginger, letting the broccoli stay as green as possible. Add it to the pumpkin. Drain the seaweed and add it to the mixture, along with most of the coriander (cilantro).

Place the mixture on a large plate and, using a metal cheese slicer, very finely slice the coconut over the vegetables. Garnish with the remaining coriander and chilli and serve immediately.

Puy Lentils with Fresh Herbs

Lentils are a rich source of minerals that benefit nearly every organ and gland in the body. They are high in protein, easily digestible and an excellent source of both magnesium and potassium – which makes them extremely helpful for balancing blood-sugar levels and thereby enhancing sleep.

3oz/90g/¾ cup Puy lentils
¼ bulb garlic, divided into cloves, trimmed and peeled
2 tbsp extra-virgin olive oil
juice of ½ lemon
2–3 tbsp fresh herbs, such as basil, marjoram, mint or oregano, finely chopped
sea salt and freshly ground black pepper

Wash the lentils and place them in a large saucepan. Cover with plenty of cold water, add the garlic in whole cloves and bring to the boil. Simmer very gently for about 20 minutes or until the lentils are just cooked. Drain, discarding the garlic. Toss the lentils in the olive oil and lemon juice. Stir in the herbs and season to taste. Serve warm with rye bread and a simple salad.

Sweet Potato and Carrot Soup

Sweet potatoes and carrots are both high in beta-carotene and vitamin C, which are important in reducing stress and thereby promoting sleep. Turmeric contains curcuminoids, anti-inflammatory compounds, which, together with cardamom (a relation of the ginger family) and coriander, will soothe and relax the digestive system. Due to the stimulatory effect of some of the herbs and spices, this soup is best consumed at lunchtime.

3 tbsp/¼C extra-virgin olive oil
3oz/85g/¾C diced carrots
3oz/85g/½C diced orange-fleshed sweet potato
2½oz/75g/½C chopped onion
5 green cardamom seeds
1 level tsp coriander seeds
2 dried bay leaves
1 level tsp turmeric
2 tsp lemon juice
7oz/200g/1¾C tomatoes, skinned and chopped
8 fl oz/250ml/1¾C vegetable stock
2 tbsp/2½ tbsp live organic yoghurt (optional)
handful of fresh chives, chopped (optional)

In a heavy saucepan heat the oil and cook the carrot, sweet potato and onion for 3 minutes. Add the spices and stir them into the oil and vegetables for 1 minute. Add the lemon juice, tomatoes and stock and simmer, covered, for 30 minutes or until the vegetables are tender. Remove the bay leaves and liquidize the contents of the pan in a food processor or blender.

This is a thick soup, but if you prefer it a bit thinner, add a little more stock at this stage and adjust the seasoning with more lemon juice and some black pepper. Serve either hot or cold, garnished with a dollop of yoghurt into which some chives have been whisked.

Lentil Soup with Mint

Lentils are rich in calcium and magnesium to help provide a good night's sleep. Adding spinach towards the end of cooking provides a valuable source of vitamin C and iron, for immune and hormonal support. Mint is a soothing balm for the entire digestive tract.

3oz/90g/½C dried lentils
1 tbsp/1½ tbsp olive oil
2 cloves garlic, minced
4oz/125g/1½C finely chopped leeks
1 level tsp dried thyme
1 level tsp dried sage
2oz/60g/½C diced parsnips
2pt/1.1l/5C water
1 tomato, skinned and chopped
4oz/115g fresh spinach, finely chopped
3 heaped tbsp fresh mint, finely chopped
1 tbsp/1½ tbsp fresh lemon juice
1 tbsp/ 1½ tbsp red wine (optional)
1 tbsp/1½ tbsp tamari or rich soy sauce
freshly ground pepper

Rinse the lentils and set them aside to drain. Heat the oil in a large soup pot. Add the garlic and leeks, then cook over a high heat for 3–4 minutes. Stir in the herbs and parsnips. Continue to sauté for 5 minutes, stirring frequently. Toss in the lentils and cook for another minute or so. Add the water. Bring to a simmer, stir in the tomatoes and partially cover the pot with a lid. Simmer for 1 hour.

Add the spinach, most of the mint, the lemon juice and the wine (if desired). Cook for 5 minutes, removing the pan from the heat just as the spinach becomes bright green. Season to taste with tamari or soy sauce and pepper. Garnish with the remaining mint.

Bean Soup with Spring Greens

Beans help to control insulin and blood-sugar levels, which is important for proper sleep and dealing with stress, while spring greens contain high levels of magnesium, as well as vitamin E.

2oz/50g/⅓C uncooked haricot beans (navy beans), soaked in water overnight
2in/5cm piece of dried kombu seaweed
4oz/115g/3C spring greens, shredded
1–2 cloves garlic, finely chopped
1 tbsp/1½ tbsp extra-virgin olive oil
sea salt and pepper

Drain the beans of their soaking water, then add some fresh water to a level about 2in/5cm above the beans, before cooking them in a heavy saucepan with the kombu. Cover and simmer the beans until soft (about 1–1½ hours). Reserve one-quarter of the beans and blend the rest with 7 fl oz/200ml/1C of the cooking liquid to make a thick purée.

In a separate pan, simmer the spring greens over a high heat in a little water for about 2 minutes, keeping them crisp. Add some of the greens' water to the soup to get the desired consistency.

In another pan gently sweat the garlic in half of the olive oil. Add it with the greens and the reserved beans to the soup and season to taste. Ladle into soup bowls and add a swirl of olive oil for aromatic flavouring. Serve at once.

Double-Artichoke Soup

Both Jerusalem (sunchokes) and globe artichokes store their carbohydrates as inulin rather than sugar, a starch that is not utilized by the body for energy, but does provide nutrition for health-promoting bacteria in the intestine. It has an insulin-like action on the body and has been shown to control blood-sugar levels – vital for balancing moods and promoting a good night's sleep.

2 medium-sized globe artichokes
½ lemon
4oz/125g Jerusalem artichokes (sunchokes)
2 tbsp/2½ tbsp extra-virgin olive oil
1 medium-sized onion, finely chopped
13 fl oz/375ml/1⅔C vegetable stock
sprig of fresh thyme
2 heaped tbsp Parmesan cheese, freshly grated

Prepare the globe artichokes by removing the tough outer leaves, then cut off the tops of the remaining leaves. Pare the stalks down to the paler tender part. Rub all the cut edges with the lemon surface to prevent discoloration. Cut the trimmed artichokes into quarters and scrape away the inner choke. Slice the quarters lengthwise into small pieces.

Peel the Jerusalem artichokes (sunchokes) and cut them into thin slices. Heat most of the olive oil and add the onion, frying gently until golden. Add the prepared artichokes and cook, stirring constantly, for about 5 minutes. Add the stock and thyme and simmer, covered, until the artichokes are tender (about 40 minutes). Serve the soup with a drizzle of olive oil and the Parmesan grated on top. It is particularly good with crostini (see p.124) – toasted Italian bread rubbed with raw garlic.

Creamy Baked Red Peppers

Red peppers are a good source of B vitamins, which helps to relax the brain and nervous system as well as aiding digestion, which is important for restful sleep. Brown rice is high in tryptophan and is also packed with the important B vitamins, while peas help to balance blood-sugar levels.

- 8oz/225g/1C short-grain brown rice
- 2 large or 4 small red peppers
- 2 tbsp/2½ tbsp extra-virgin olive oil
- 1 small onion, finely chopped
- 2 cloves garlic, finely chopped
- medium handful of sunflower seeds
- 2oz/50g/½C green peas, fresh or frozen, blanched and refreshed in cold water
- 2oz/50g/¼C low-fat cottage cheese
- 2 heaped tsp finely chopped fresh parsley
- 30g/1oz/⅓C grated Parmesan cheese
- salt and pepper

Put the rice in a saucepan with twice its volume of cold water and cover. Bring to the boil, turn down to a simmer and cook until all the water has disappeared (about 40 minutes). Meanwhile, preheat the oven to 350°F/180°C/gas mark 4. Prepare the peppers by carefully slicing off the tops (keeping them intact) and removing and discarding the seeds and pith. Put all the peppers to one side.

Heat the olive oil in a pan and gently fry the onion and garlic until they are a pale golden brown, taking care not to burn them. Add the cooked rice and sunflower seeds, stirring gently for a few minutes to coat them. Remove the pan from the heat and gently mix in the peas, cottage cheese, parsley and Parmesan. Season to taste.

Stuff the peppers with the rice mixture and replace the tops. Place them tightly together, standing up on a baking dish, with ¼in/5mm of water in the bottom to steam them. Bake in the oven for 35–45 minutes (depending on size) and serve immediately.

Lemon Chicken with Sage

As well as being a lean source of high-quality protein, chicken is high in chromium – one of the most important minerals for balancing blood-sugar levels, therefore promoting sound sleep.

8oz/250g chicken breast, skin and bones removed
2fl oz/50ml/¼C vegetable stock or bouillon
1 heaped tsp black peppercorns
2 heaped tbsp chopped fresh sage leaves
zest and juice of ½ lemon
3 tbsp/½C thick plain yoghurt
salt and pepper

Cut the chicken into thin strips. Heat the stock in a wok or heavy saucepan. Add the chicken strips and gently poach them with the peppercorns, sage and lemon zest. Cook over a medium heat for 3 minutes.

Using a slotted spoon, remove the chicken from the pan. Turn up the heat and boil to reduce the stock by a quarter. Remove from the heat, then add the yoghurt and lemon juice. Put the chicken back into the pan and stir to coat it. Taste the sauce and season with salt and pepper. Serve with steamed spring greens and thick rice noodles.

Warm Vegetable Salad with Herb Dressing

Broccoli, cauliflower and even Brussels sprouts are suitable for this recipe – all are rich in the important minerals calcium and magnesium, helping to combat stress and relax the body.

5oz/150g broccoli florets
5oz/150g cauliflower florets
2 rashers organic rindless bacon (optional), cut into small pieces

For the dressing:
handful of fresh flat-leaf (Italian) parsley
handful of fresh mint
handful of fresh basil
1 clove garlic, roughly chopped
1tsp Dijon mustard
2 tbsp/2½ tbsp extra-virgin olive oil
1 tbsp/1½ tbsp lemon juice
salt and freshly ground black pepper

Bring a large pan of water to the boil and cook the florets for about 4 minutes, until tender but still firm. Drain and keep warm. Cook the bacon (if desired) in a frying pan in its own fat until crisp, then drain off the fat onto some kitchen roll.

To make the dressing, put the parsley, mint, basil, garlic and mustard in a food processor or blender. Pulse lightly and add the olive oil in a steady stream. Add the lemon juice and season to taste.

Place the broccoli and cauliflower on a serving dish. Pour over the dressing and toss gently to coat. Sprinkle the bacon over the top and serve at once.

Honeyed Prawn or Shrimp Kebabs

Prawns (shrimp) are an abundant source of zinc and magnesium, both major stress-busters, as well as selenium, a vital antioxidant for reversing damage to the cells in our bodies caused by excess stress.

2 tbsp/2½ tbsp sesame oil
2 tbsp/2½ tbsp honey
2 tbsp/2½ tbsp Dijon mustard
1 tbsp/1½ tbsp tamari or rich soy sauce
1 tbsp/1½ tbsp lemon juice
1lb/500g medium prawns (shrimp)
8oz/250g vegetables of your choice, such as onions, mushrooms, courgettes (zucchini), peppers and squash, cut into cubes

Preheat the grill. Mix the oil, honey, mustard, tamari or soy sauce and lemon juice together in a large bowl. Taste and adjust the seasoning if desired. Peel, de-vein and rinse the prawns (shrimp), then toss them in the marinade. Leave in the refrigerator for 15–60 minutes.

Thread the prawns (shrimp) onto skewers, alternating each one with a vegetable. Leave a small space between so that the prawns (shrimp) cook evenly. Put the skewers in a baking dish and pour the remaining marinade over them. Grill for 5 minutes, turning occasionally until the prawns (shrimp) become orange. Serve with rice or pasta and a green salad.

Lazy chicken pot

This is a very simple, yet delicious, dish that requires only a few minutes of preparation.

1 medium-sized onion
4 fl oz/100ml/½C extra-virgin olive oil
2 carrots
1 parsnip
1 sweet potato
1 medium-sized chicken
3½pt/2l/9C boiling water
2 heaped tbsp powdered vegetable stock or bouillon
½oz/15g cornflour (cornstarch)
4 sprigs fresh lemon thyme

Preheat the oven to 350°F/180°C/gas mark 4.

Chop the onion and place it with the olive oil in a casserole, large enough to hold the chicken, over a medium heat. Cook the onion until it is translucent. Meanwhile peel the other vegetables and cut them into small chunks. Add them to the casserole and combine with the onion. Now add the entire chicken, having first removed any giblets.

Cover with the water, then add the stock. Mix the cornflour (cornstarch) with a little cold water and combine well, then add it to the casserole with the lemon thyme. Put the lid on the casserole, or cover with foil, and place in the oven for an hour and a half.

Stir-Fried Tofu with Cashew Nuts

Tofu and cashew nuts provide excellent levels of magnesium, calcium and vegetable protein for balancing blood-sugar levels and inducing a good night's sleep. Tofu also contains phyto-oestrogens, which help to balance the hormones – a hormonal imbalance being one cause of sleep disturbances. In addition. the nuts contain zinc, another mineral for benefiting the nervous system and combating stress – a common cause of insomnia. The vegetables are abundant in magnesium, calcium and vitamin C, all vital stress-busters, and rich in B vitamins that support the nervous system.

2 tbsp/2½ tbsp extra-virgin olive oil
4oz/115g/1C firm, organic tofu, cubed
1 small onion, finely chopped
2 cloves garlic
1 small green or red pepper, chopped
1 heaped tsp fresh ginger root, grated
1 stick celery, chopped
1 courgette (zucchini), chopped
2 small carrots, sliced
4oz/125g/4C thinly sliced spring cabbage
handful of cashew nuts
5 mushrooms, wiped and sliced
8 fl oz/250ml/1C vegetable stock or bouillon
1 tbsp/1½ tbsp tamari or rich soy sauce
3 heaped tbsp chopped fresh coriander (cilantro)

Heat the oil in a wok or heavy frying pan, add the tofu cubes and fry lightly until golden brown. Remove with a spoon and place on one side. Sauté the onion, garlic, green or red pepper, ginger, celery and courgette (zucchini) over a medium heat until soft but not brown. Add the carrots, cabbage and cashew nuts, sauté for 3–4 minutes, then add the mushrooms and sauté for a further minute. Add the stock, return the tofu to the pan, cover and steam until the vegetables are soft but still have bite (about 3 minutes). Season with tamari or soy sauce to taste, sprinkle with the coriander (cilantro) and serve with a grain of your choice.

Vegetable Stew with Pistou

This light, juicy stew provides a full gamut of nutrients, especially calcium and magnesium to encourage sleep, and fibre (from the vegetables), which is important for good digestion. The pine nuts provide an excellent source of protein to help balance blood-sugar levels.

2 tbsp/2½ tbsp extra-virgin olive oil
1 medium-sized onion, cut into quarters
3 cloves garlic, roughly chopped
2oz/50g/scant ½C roughly chopped carrot
3oz/85g/¾C roughly chopped potato
2oz/50g/½C celery, cut into 1in/2.5cm pieces
3 medium-sized tomatoes, skinned and chopped
5fl oz/150ml/⅔C vegetable stock or bouillon
salt and pepper

For the pistou:
4 heaped tbsp roughly chopped basil
2 tbsp/¼C pine nuts, finely chopped
1 clove garlic, crushed
1 tbsp/1½ tbsp extra-virgin olive oil

Heat the oven to 350°F/180°C/gas mark 4. In a heavy cooking pot heat the olive oil over a medium heat and add the onion. Cook for 2 minutes until the onion is well coated with oil and beginning to soften. Add the garlic and cook for a minute longer. Add the rest of the vegetables, stirring to coat them thoroughly in the oil. Add the stock, cover the pot with a lid and place in the oven for 1 hour.

Meanwhile prepare the pistou by mixing the basil, pine nuts and garlic together with the oil until it makes a paste.

Check that the vegetables in the stew are tender and season to taste. Place the stew on individual warm plates or in bowls, add a spoonful of pistou and swirl it in. Serve with wild rice and a simple green salad.

Pineapple, Raspberry and Lime Ice

Pineapple contains bromelain, a protein-digesting enzyme with immense power, so it is generally helpful for digestive complaints which may cause sleeplessness. It also helps clear mucous waste from the bronchial tissues and may therefore alleviate conditions such as snoring and sleep apnoea. Raspberries are also a good cleanser of catarrhal conditions.

4oz/125g/1C chopped fresh pineapple
4oz/125g/¾C raspberries, fresh or frozen
3 tbsp/¼C lime juice
1 tbsp/1½ tbsp honey
1 heaped tbsp grated lime zest
2 fl oz/50ml/¼C water
sprigs of fresh mint or slices of lime, to garnish

In a blender or food processor, blend together all the ingredients except the garnish. Strain the blended liquid, discarding any pulp from the pineapple and seeds from the raspberries, then pour the thick juice into a bowl and place in the freezer.

After 2–3 hours remove from the freezer and break the ice into large chunks. Blend again in the food processor until smooth and creamy. Return to the freezer for at least another 30 minutes before serving.

To serve, scoop the fruit ice onto serving plates or into tall glasses. Garnish with sprigs of fresh mint or slices of lime.

Fig and Apricot Whip

Dried figs have one of the highest calcium contents of any food in the plant world, and apricots are also an excellent source. Figs are also high in the amino acid tryptophan, which promotes sleep. The Greek yoghurt provides important protein for balancing blood-sugar levels and beneficial bacteria for easing digestive complaints that could interrupt sleep patterns.

2oz/60g/½C dried figs
2oz/60g/½C dried apricots
5 fl oz/150ml/⅔C water
½ tbsp apple-juice concentrate
½ tbsp lemon juice
1 tbsp/1½ tbsp honey
2 tbsp/⅓C thick organic Greek yoghurt
sprinkling of nutmeg
1 heaped tbsp flaked almonds

Wash the figs and apricots. Mix the water with the apple-juice concentrate, lemon juice and honey. Pour the mixture over the figs and apricots and leave to soak, covered, overnight.

Put the fruit mixture in a pan, bring to the boil and simmer until soft (about 5–10 minutes). Leave to cool, then purée. Spoon the pudding into individual dishes, top with a generous dollop of Greek yoghurt, a dusting of nutmeg and a few flaked almonds.

Banana and Chocolate Mousse

A rich-tasting, smooth pudding without any dairy products! As an occasional treat, this delicious dessert is packed full of magnesium, both from the tofu (which makes it creamy) and from the chocolate (which makes it so delicious). Tofu is also high in calcium, which – combined with the magnesium – will help promote a good night's sleep. Bananas are high in the amino acid tryptophan, a natural sleep inducer, and therefore a perfect late-night treat.

1oz/30g/¼ cup dark chocolate, 70 per cent cocoa
6oz/170g/1¼ C tofu, cubed
1 large ripe banana, chopped
½ tsp vanilla extract
2 tbsp/2½ tbsp honey
pinch of salt
1 tsp raspberry vinegar

Melt the chocolate carefully in a double boiler, or in a Pyrex bowl set over gently boiling water. Remove from the heat.

Place the tofu and half the banana in a blender and begin to purée it. Gradually add the remaining banana, pulsing it between additions to make sure that it whips up smoothly. Add the vanilla, honey, salt and raspberry vinegar as you go. Pour in the melted chocolate. Purée the mixture again until it is very smooth. Taste for sweetness, adding either more honey or vinegar as necessary. Transfer it to a large bowl or individual serving dishes, cover tightly and chill for at least 2 hours before serving.

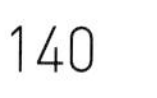

Sesame-Seed Dip

Sesame seeds are high in zinc, calcium, magnesium and the amino acid tryptophan – all wonderful nutrients for coping with stress and encouraging restful sleep.

2oz/60g/½C sesame seeds
8 fl oz/250ml/1C Greek yoghurt
1–2 tbsp/1½–2½ tbsp tamari or rich soy sauce

Dry-roast the sesame seeds in a frying pan set over a moderate heat, until they start to pop and are barely browned. Transfer them to a bowl and allow to cool. Stir in the yoghurt and tamari, then spoon the dip into a small bowl.

Babaganouj

Aubergines (eggplants) have a soothing and stabilizing effect on the nervous system, as well as being high in calcium to encourage good sleep. This pâté has a cleansing effect on the body.

2 medium-sized aubergines (eggplants)
2oz/50g/¼C tahini paste
juice of 1 lemon
3 heaped tbsp finely chopped fresh parsley
pinch of sea salt
1 tsp extra-virgin olive oil (optional)

Preheat the oven to 400°F/205°C/gas mark 6. Prick the aubergines (eggplants) with a fork, place them in a roasting dish in the oven and bake until slightly charred and bursting (about 45 minutes). Remove from the oven and allow to cool completely.

Cut the aubergines (eggplants) in half, scoop out the flesh and mash well or purée in a food processor or blender. Combine with the tahini, lemon juice, parsley and sea salt. Check the seasoning. Drizzle some olive oil over the top before serving (if desired). Serve with a selection of crudités, such as carrot, cucumber and celery sticks, broccoli and cauliflower florets and/or warmed pitta bread.

Other sleep-inducing snacks

- Cottage cheese with basil and alfalfa on pumpernickel bread
- Tofu dip, made from mixing tofu with ground sesame/sunflower seeds and miso
- Mashed banana and sesame-seed paste (tahini) on Ryvita
- Date and banana smoothie (1 banana and 3 dates mixed with 1C of soya milk and blended).

a note on measurements

This book uses metric, Imperial and American measurements. Dry ingredients are meansured in ounces/grams, ounces/grams/US cups, Imperial spoons/US spoons or Imperial spoons/US cups. Liquid ingredients are measured either in Imperial fluid ounces/millilitres/US cups (1 Imperial pint = 20 fluid ounces = 0.568 litre; 1 US pint = 16 fluid ounces = 0.550 litre) or Imperial spoons/US cups or Imperial spoons/US spoons.

The recipes refer to Imperial pints as used in the UK and Australia which contain 20 fl oz. The American pint contains 16 fl oz. Cups refer to the US 8 fl oz measuring cup. A teaspoon is standard at approximately 5ml, however tablespoons do vary. The measures in this book refer to the UK standard (17.7ml) and the American standard (14.2ml). The tables below gives a conversion chart:

UK	US	Australian
17.7ml	14.2ml	20ml
1 tablespoon	1 tablespoon	1 tablespoon
2 tablespoons	3 tablespoons	2 tablespoons
3½ tablespoons	4 tablespoons	3 tablespoons
4 tablespoons	5 tablespoons	3½ tablespoons

useful addresses

UK ORGANIZATIONS

British Association for Counselling and Psychotherapy
1 Regents Close
Rugby
Warwickshire CV21 2PJ
tel. 0870 443 5252
www.bac.co.uk

The British Nutrition Foundation
52–54 High Holborn
London WC1V 6RQ
tel. 020 7404 6504
www.nutrition.org.uk

The Institute for Optimum Nutrition
Blades Court
Deodar Road
London SW15 2NU
tel. 020 8877 9993
www.ion.ac.uk

The Sleep Council
High Corn Mill
Chapel Hill
Skipton
North Yorkshire BD23 1NL
tel. 01756 791089
www.sleepcouncil.org.uk

Women's Nutritional Advisory Service
PO Box 268
Lewes
Sussex BN7 2QN
tel. 01273 487366
www.wnas.org.uk

US ORGANIZATIONS

American Association for World Health
1825 K Street, NW, Suite 1208
Washington DC 20006
tel. 202-466-5883
www.aawhworldhealth.org

American Counselling Association
5999 Stevenson Avenue
Alexandria
VI 22304-3300
tel. 703-823-9800
www.counselling.org

Food Allergy Network
10400 Eaton Place, ste. 107
Fairfax, VA 22030-2208
tel. 800-929-4040
www.foodallergy.org

National Institute of Nutritional Education
1010 S. Joliet 107
Aurora, CO 80012
tel. 800-530-8079
www.ahsu.com

National Sleep Foundation
1522 K Street, NW, Suite 500
Washington DC 20005
tel. 202-347-3471
www.sleepfoundation.org

general index

For recipes, see recipe index on page 144.

recipe index